MEDICAL FASCISM

HOW CORONAVIRUS POLICY
TOOK OUR FREEDOMS AWAY
AND HOW TO GET THEM BACK

ROB RYDER

Copyright © Rob Ryder 2021
All Rights Reserved.
This book is sold subject to the condition that it shall not, by way of trade or otherwise, be lent, resold, hired out, or otherwise circulated without the publisher's prior consent in any form of binding or cover other than that in which it is published and without a similar condition including this condition being imposed on the subsequent publisher.
The moral right of Rob Ryder has been asserted.
ISBN: 9798514158577

This book has not been created to be specific to any individual's or organizations' situation or needs. Every effort has been made to make this book as accurate as possible. This book should serve only as a general guide and not as the ultimate source of subject information. This book contains information that might be dated and is intended only to educate and entertain. The author shall have no liability or responsibility to any person or entity regarding any loss or damage incurred, or alleged to have incurred, directly or indirectly, by the information contained in this book.

This book is dedicated to historians and their pursuit of Truth, Justice, and Freedom – who have kept alive the knowledge of the true nature of human beings and suffered ridicule, injustice, and even death to set a foundation and example as mankind enters the "end times".

ACKNOWLEDGEMENTS

There are too many people to thank for helping me with my research and giving me the opportunity and help to follow my chosen path. Most of you know who you are and get a mention in the book. So I would just like to thank one person, my mother, for setting an example for work ethic, not feeling sorry for yourself, not being a victim, giving an example of how to be the best person you can within the circumstances put in front of you, and always putting your kids first.

"Taking the information coming out of the official covid-19 narrative the author reconnects it to other aspects of how the medical authorities have been consistently ignoring science. He links it to the position of power the owners of the medical profession occupy within governments and within the financial system. It appears they can afford to lie and to deceive the public and not only are they getting away unscathed but they are even being rewarded for it. The author confirms that the only way this system of complete control over the population can be broken is for the population to make independent free choices. And for this to happen we all need this information."

- Dr Patrick Quanten

CONTENTS

DECLARATION 1
INTRODUCTION 3
HEALTH 5
   What is it to be healthy? 5
SYMPTOMS OF ILLNESS 7
   Body gone wrong – body doing right? 7
   GP – body malfunctions 7
   Homeopath – body rebalances 7
   The Germ or The Soil 8
   Louis Pasteur, 1822-1894 – Germ Theory 8
   Antoine Béchamp, 1816-1908 – Soil Theory 8
   Consequences 9
   Homeopath 9
   Koch's Postulates 10
   Infection 13
   Redness – pain – swelling – heat 14
   Viruses 14
   Polio 18
   DDT 21
   Antivirals 23
BALANCE 24
VACCINATION ON TRIAL 27
    Reality 28
    Boosters 35
    Possible scenario 36
    Data not widely published 37
    Unclear dates on graphs 37
    Measles 38
    Fraud 44
    Notes on letter 48
    Law of Consent 49
    Defining consent 49
    Watch YouTube – "The Fluoride Deception" 53
THE HISTORY OF MODERN MEDICINE 58
    Toxic takeover 59
    Toxic Psychiatry 62
    Legacy of Modern Medicine 66
    Bill & Melinda Gates Foundation 67

"Transact in the modern world"	73
MEDICAL DOCTORS	77
THE GLOBAL PANDEMIC – WHAT JUST HAPPENED?	80
EVENT 201 – YOUTUBE "Event 201 Pandemic Exercise"	80
Note	87
THE SCIENTIFIC METHOD	88
Dr Andrew Kaufman	89
Reliability of antibody and PCR tests	92
My notes	92
Statement On Virus Isolation (SOVI)	96
THE FIRST WAVE	97
Italy	97
Lombardy	97
Spain	101
Terrorism ACT200	103
The Enemy Has Landed	104
Professor Neil Ferguson – Imperial College London	108
Enter the "77th brigade"	116
DEATH BY LOCKDOWN?	119
Care home deaths	120
Hospital deaths	125
Community deaths	127
Conclusions	128
UK Column	129
Death from anxiety	134
Sweden	135
Japan	138
Peru	140
USA	141
Mask Madness – Mask Murder	142
Clean hands please	144
Summer on the beach	144
SECOND WAVE OF MADNESS	147
IT'S ALL A MIND GAME	156
Perception	160
Suffer Little Children	165
THE WAR ON INFORMATION AND TRUTH	169
THE SYSTEM	172
Human Sovereignty	172
The Freeman Movement	172
Society	172

- Public servants or leaders? 174
- Compromise Yes, Conform No 174
- Just say NO 174
- Police State 175

FOLLOW THE MONEY 177
- Central Banks 179
- Glass Steagall 180
- The myth of a gold-backed currency 181
- A just monetary system for all 182
- Beware the Gobal Reset – World Economic Forum 184

WHAT NEXT? 187
- Action 189
- The pen is mightier than the sword 189
- It's now a spiritual battle 191

THE BEST CHICKEN SOUP EVER! 194

DECLARATION

My name is Robert Ryder. To start, you must know I am not a "medical expert" and am not trained in medical science. I am just a simple guy who has been researching life, how it works, health and disease and world events for about 15 years. I do, though, have an O Level in English and maths, which in the system we live in, means I am qualified to read and understand the English language and understand and interpret simple maths and data, including graphs.

In about 2011, I saw an interview on alternative TV with medical biochemist Trevor Gunn that blew me away with the simplicity of what he was saying. I needed to know more. I immediately bought his book, *The Science of Health and Healing*, which then forced me to rethink everything I thought was true about the nature of disease. This book is the culmination of my work and research and should not be considered as truth at face value. Do your own research. It is also not to be taken as medical advice. Accident and emergency aside, I do not use modern medicine, but in any situation you should take advice from those who you trust and in the end make your own decision and stand by it. This book should be taken purely for what it is, information. What you make of it is up to you; it is your life, after all, and your life is not my responsibility, something that will become clearer after reading this book.

I am also not a professional author and don't even have good computer skills, so any messy writing or simple errors should be excused. It's the information that counts, not my style. I have tried my best to produce a presentable piece of work that many can understand; after that, it is what it is. The book has been influenced by many great people whose work gets a mention.

Like the great Australian Max Igan said: **"If I used your work it's because it was the best."**

Robert Ryder, March 2021

All Rights Reserved

"Believe nothing, no matter where you read it, or who said it, no matter if I have said it, unless it agrees with your own reason and your own common sense."

– Buddha allegedly

INTRODUCTION

I am writing this book in the middle of goings-on that are really something out of a science-fiction film.

This is a scenario that I knew was going to happen in some form for many years; I never knew exactly how but I knew it would happen. I knew when the propaganda first started coming out of China that this could well come over here and go worldwide, in fact my friend and I warned about this before it landed here[1], so I was kind of prepared, but when the news finally came out – "we are going into lockdown" – it felt very surreal. Obviously, there was confusion with most people, others just thought that this would be over in a couple of weeks and life would go back to "normal" and sadly others were terrified of this invisible enemy coming to get them, coming to get all of us. I knew straight away that it wasn't going to pass over and that this was it, it was finally happening. The end battle for humanity's freedom is now underway and possibly within a year the outcome will be an absolute slavery we will never get out of, or an incredible freedom which will finally give humanity the chance to see what it can really do.

Information is changing on a daily basis so I'm not even sure what the world will be like, or what new truths will be unveiled, or what the latest version of events will be by the time it is finished, so this is my best effort with the information I have at the present time to show you what is happening and why. I am not claiming my version of events is truth, but it is my truth. I have been diligent in my research but cannot say for sure that anything is absolute fact; fake news comes from all areas, especially governments and medical science, but my interpretation of the information is my own and it is for all of us to interpret as truthfully as we can regardless of what anyone else thinks, or what the crowd says, or especially what the government tells us.

There is too much information, so I have tried to put together individual pieces to show that it makes a bigger, interconnected picture. It is then up to the individual to research and put more pieces of the puzzle in and

---

[1] https://www.youtube.com/watch?v=kawc3tBUo2Q

see what the end picture tells them. Whether you come to the same conclusions as me is up to you; as you will see, perceiving the world and information is a very individual thing, but I know the best place to start is from a blank page.

To find truth is like looking for a needle in a haystack; the only way to do it is to first discard the hay (untruths) and what is left over will be the needle (truth).

HEALTH

What is it to be healthy?

First, we have to understand that we are all individuals, so for example a man of 5 feet 8 inches may weigh ten stones and have a different blood pressure and other things to a man of the same height but who weighs 14 stones. Maybe one is a runner, the other a rugby player, both physically fit for their build and lifestyle. So based on somebody's height it would be impossible to tell someone their perfect weight, blood pressure, etc., as we are all different. Also, health cannot be defined by lack of symptoms, just as illness cannot be defined by the presence of symptoms. An example could be a fever; the body needs energy and vitality to produce a fever so the presence of a fever to burn up unhealthy tissues could be a sign of good health, healthy maintenance, whereas a person who cannot produce a fever could be loaded up with toxins, struggling to expel them.

There are basic things a human needs to be healthy, which include having the body parts/organs in good working order, clean blood, a clean and healthy environment with sunlight and fresh air, living free from enforced stress, good nutrition, and to be completely aware and in control of who you are, freely expressing yourself. The sign of good health is known as vitality, the vital force that powers our cells. This we take from the energy source that is the sun, breathing clean fresh air and being true to ourselves and expressing our true individualism. Signs of vitality are people who are creative, happy, alert, heal quickly and have a thirst for life. Lack of vitality could include depression, fatigue, low energy, slow healing and no sense of purpose. As science has shown we are all energy at our source; our physical bodies are perfect expressions of our true energetic selves. Think of that when someone asks why they have cancer and the doctor just says, "Bad luck."

So, health could be best described as an individual being in balance with him/herself and the world he/she finds themselves in, living a life with purpose and following dreams and embracing the great game of life, and as we are all different – we like different foods, climates, lifestyles and have different personalities – we need to find our own personal balance. So, if health is being in balance then sickness could be described as being out of balance, not being or expressing your true self.

We will now delve into some theories of how we go from one state to the other. Please leave any preconceived ideas at one side and start with a blank page, and go with the evidence and what feels right for you. After all, the responsibility for your health is your own. In my opinion the main things needed for health are clean water, sunshine, fresh air, family and friends and a sense of purpose. These are the very things the lockdown has taken away from people in the name of health, not a coincidence in my opinion.

SYMPTOMS OF ILLNESS

Body gone wrong – body doing right?

When we are ill we become aware of this as the body produces symptoms like fever, vomiting and rashes, etc., or just a feeling of being unwell. But what do these symptoms mean? Compare the view of your GP and, say, a homeopath.

GP – body malfunctions

Trained in allopathic thinking, so symptoms like a fever a rash, headache, and inflammation are seen as the body going wrong. Very little time is spent on asking why this has come about, only that it is a discomfort to you and it needs to be fixed. Therefore, the doctor will look at his list of drugs to find one that will stop or suppress the symptom, as they see the symptom as the problem. So by taking away the discomfort (symptom) the patient feels well and believes all is fine again. Though doctors are aware that fevers are getting rid of cellular waste and toxicity, they still treat this as the problem most of the time, the body going wrong, a malfunction, part of a broken machine not knowing what it is doing. They normally get about ten minutes with patients, only enough time to look at symptoms.

Homeopath – body rebalances

They are trained in seeing the body when showing symptoms of illness, as the body trying to re-establish health, and view symptoms, or patterns of symptoms, as an intelligent reaction by the body to try and bring back balance, basically a clearing-out of bad stuff. Therefore, they prescribe safe remedies that aid the body with whatever symptom is being shown, going with the body, kind of giving the body a helping hand, going with the intelligence of the body and trusting that the body knows what is best. After all, it has had plenty of time to evolve and perfect these responses.

They normally give the patient an hour to listen and put together a holistic view of what's going on in that particular life.

The Germ or The Soil

> **"The specific disease doctrine is the grand refuge of weak, uncultured, unstable minds, such as now rule in the medical profession. There are no specific diseases; there are specific disease conditions."**
>
> – Florence Nightingale

Louis Pasteur, 1822-1894 – Germ Theory

A 'survival of the fittest' view. Microbes came about and decided to attack and invade us from the outside. Microbes are non-changeable (monomorphism), they cause disease, each microbe with its own specific disease and symptoms. Solution: kill or avoid the microbe.

Antoine Béchamp, 1816-1908 – Soil Theory

A harmonious view. Microbes, or the potential for microbes (microzymas), are in all living things and evolve into different forms – bacteria, fungi, etc. – depending on the soil (pleomorphism). Toxicity of the soil causes disease, and then microbes associated with the terrain will be seen. Their birthplace is from within the diseased tissue and not from outside, so they are not the cause but the result of toxicity of the soil. Like worms in a composter they are part of the cleaning up process. Solution is to address the terrain (soil), look at diet, lifestyle, environment, stress, etc., and makes the needed changes to support the body in healing.

Consequences

GP

Microbes are to blame for infections, therefore we need a silver bullet to kill the invader. Symptoms are the body malfunctioning so we need drugs to stop the process. So we have the birth of Big Pharma with suppressive drugs like anti-biotics, anti-inflammatories, anti-histamines and others. Governments and big corporations don't have to worry about the environment and social conditions. Most importantly, people are not responsible for their own health and no lifestyle changes are needed, we are just random victims, we live in fear of microbes and our bodies have no ability to self-heal, hence we become dependent on doctors and their corporate drugs.

Homeopath

Lifestyle, diet, emotional state, mental state and all aspects of the environment are things to look at for a full understanding of a life out of balance that has led to toxicity in the body and illness. No need for Big Pharma drugs and vaccines. Governments and big corporations need to keep the environment clean, raise social standards and organise a less stressful society. Most importantly YOU are responsible for your own health and it is YOUR responsibility when you get ill.

> **"If I could live my life over again, I would devote it to proving that germs seek their natural habitat – diseased tissue – rather than being the cause of dead tissue."**
> – Dr Rudolf Virchow, the Father of Modern Pathology

Even during the times of Louis Pasteur, his germ theory of disease was not held by the entire scientific community. I recommend a book by Henry Lindlahr MD, *Nature Cure*, published in 1914, for his extensive knowledge and research into disease and criticism of Pasteur and allopathic thinking. In the book he quoted another doctor at the time who had travelled the world and came back with the conclusion that cancer is a disease of modern living. He also noted how in his practices he had cured all diseases with natural, simple treatments mainly focusing on rest, simple foods, sunlight and breathing exercises and always working with the body and not against it. An article by Patrick Quanten MD goes into a simple history of the battle of ideas between Pasteur and Béchamp.[2]

As you will see later on, things like clean water and sanitation and better living conditions were what caused the massive drop in infectious disease at the turn of the century and not vaccination programmes, backing up very clearly Béchamp and his soil theory. The reason the world took to Germ Theory could well be governments and big corporations not wanting to take on the costly task of looking after the people, the control over them it gave, and also that people never really want to take responsibility for their own lives. A combination of these seems about right.

Koch's Postulates

In 1890 the criteria for seeing if a given bacteria was the cause of a certain disease was put down by Robert Koch, German physician and bacteriologist.

> **The bacteria must be present in every case of the disease.**
>
> **The bacteria must be isolated from the host with the disease and grown in pure culture.**
>
> **The specific disease must be reproduced when a pure culture of the bacteria is inoculated into a healthy susceptible host.**
>
> **The bacteria must be recoverable from the experimentally infected host.**

These criteria, though before the time when we could identify viruses, could also be used to prove causation of viruses in disease. The problem they have is that many bacteria and viruses that we are told are the causes of disease are found in many people without producing any symptoms at all. Hib, meningococcal and *E. coli* bacteria we are told cause meningitis are found in healthy people, as are HPV, HIV, herpes and polio viruses (alleged viruses). So how is it possible that these are the causes of disease? Obviously these microbes have their place in our inner

---

[2] http://www.activehealthcare.co.uk/index.php/literature/medical/65-the-origin-of-germs

ecosystem; they have a job to do and for most of us don't cause a problem, so for us to find them in a disease situation, we need to ask ourselves, what changed in the body for these microbes to be associated with disease? Remember, the criteria say these microbes must be present in all cases of the disease; therefore a healthy person shouldn't have microbes we are told are the causes of disease in their system.

Why is it that bacteria or viruses we already have in us can proliferate, become invasive and cause things like meningitis? And why has it not been shown possible to infect a healthy person with a pure isolated virus and make that person ill with the associated disease?

We also know that bacteria feed off diseased cells and waste and not healthy cells. Ask any dentist why you get a gum infection and he will tell you that it's for not clearing out the food waste, or too much sugar; in other words keep the environment clean and no infection. Yes, a dentist, whether they know it or not, believes in soil theory.

As for proving the passing of viruses from person to person causing disease, this extract from an article by John M. Eyler, PhD, The State of Science, Microbiology, and Vaccines circa 1918, shows us how this was always just an unproven theory:

> "Perhaps the most interesting epidemiological studies conducted during the 1918-1919 pandemic were the human experiments conducted by the Public Health Service and the U.S. Navy under the supervision of Milton Rosenau on Gallops Island, the quarantine station in Boston Harbor, and on Angel Island, its counterpart in San Francisco. The experiment began with 100 volunteers from the Navy who had no history of influenza. Rosenau was the first to report on the experiments conducted at Gallops Island in November and December 1918. His first volunteers received first one strain and then several strains of Pfeiffer's bacillus by spray and swab into their noses and throats and then into their eyes. When that procedure failed to produce disease, others were inoculated with mixtures of other organisms isolated from the throats and noses of influenza patients. Next, some volunteers received injections of blood from influenza patients. Finally, 13 of the volunteers were taken into an influenza ward and exposed to 10 influenza patients each. Each volunteer was to shake hands with each patient, to talk with him at close range, and to permit him to cough directly into his face. None of the volunteers in these experiments developed influenza. Rosenau was clearly puzzled, and he cautioned against

drawing conclusions from negative results. He ended his article in JAMA with a telling acknowledgement: "We entered the outbreak with a notion that we knew the cause of the disease, and were quite sure we knew how it was transmitted from person to person. Perhaps, if we have learned anything, it is that we are not quite sure what we know about the disease." The research conducted at Angel Island and that continued in early 1919 in Boston broadened this research by inoculating with the Mathers streptococcus and by including a search for filter-passing agents, but it produced similar negative results. It seemed that what was acknowledged to be one of the most contagious of communicable diseases could not be transferred under experimental conditions." [3]

Even one of the deadliest pandemics known to man, the Great Spanish Flu of 1918, could not be proven to be caused by a contagious microbe. It was based on a theory borne out of Louis Pasteur and Germ Theory and they were trying to explain an outbreak of an illness without looking at all factors. The belief in a thing being the cause had taken over the minds of the medical profession; a thing, though, that they could not really see or test.

We also know that in cases of flu the symptoms can be present but in many cases no "flu virus" can be detected.

The theory had more holes than Swiss cheese, so they again had to change the science to fit the belief. When it was clear Koch's Postulates could not be used for viruses as they were too small to isolate, then new criteria was put in place.

Here are Koch's postulates for the 21st century as suggested by Fredricks and Relman:

Fredericks DN, & Relman DA (1996). Sequence-based identification of microbial pathogens: a reconsideration of Koch's postulates.

> A nucleic acid sequence belonging to a putative pathogen should be present in most cases of an infectious disease. Microbial nucleic acids should be found preferentially in those organs or gross anatomic sites known to be diseased, and not in those organs that lack pathology.

---

[3] https://www.ncbi.nlm.nih.gov/pmc/articles/PMC2862332/

Fewer, or no, copy numbers of pathogen-associated nucleic acid sequences should occur in hosts or tissues without disease.

With resolution of disease, the copy number of pathogen-associated nucleic acid sequences should decrease or become undetectable. With clinical relapse, the opposite should occur.

When sequence detection predates disease, or sequence copy number correlates with severity of disease or pathology, the sequence-disease association is more likely to be a causal relationship.

The nature of the microorganism inferred from the available sequence should be consistent with the known biological characteristics of that group of organisms.

Tissue-sequence correlates should be sought at the cellular level: efforts should be made to demonstrate specific in situ hybridization of microbial sequence to areas of tissue pathology and to visible microorganisms or to areas where microorganisms are presumed to be located.

These sequence-based forms of evidence for microbial causation should be reproducible.

With that criteria and the knowledge that many microbes and viruses are found in healthy people, it would certainly be easy to come to any conclusion that was wanted by controlling the narrative and therefore how the masses, including medical students, receive the information. The original criteria were very precise and clear and it seems we do now have the technology to purely isolate viruses. So why is it not being done?

Infection

An infection is classed as an inflammation with germs. So straight away, we see that something, inflammation, has already occurred in the body. So what is inflammation? It is said to be four things that all have to be present; if not, it can't be inflammation.

Redness – pain – swelling – heat

It would seem that if these things are happening in a particular area of the body, then that area has an issue with damaged or diseased tissue that the body is trying to heal by burning up the waste to be disposed of. So if an infection is inflammation with germs, then it is clear that the problem, diseased or damaged tissue, is already there. If, then, the inflammation is not enough and the tissue deteriorates, you may get an "infection". This is just an extra effort by the body to restore balance and from within the diseased tissue, the things we call germs emerge to feed off the waste. With this extra effort there could well then be a full-body fever and not localised heat and again, this would seem to be an extra effort to burn waste out of the body and excrete it through the skin, the main and largest detoxification organ. So although bacteria may be a part of life and around us everywhere, it's clear that to survive they need their own very specific food supply. No food means they will die, like all life, so even if you are exposed to bacteria that enter your system, if you have no food (waste), they cannot proliferate and if there is food, eventually your body would produce those same microbes itself anyway. You cannot "catch" watch you are not susceptible to.

In the case of childhood illness it has always been known that these are illnesses of development and a clearing out of the system for the child to grow and find a new balance. In a growing experience of the world and life, growth can mean change and change can mean clearing out of the system what is not functioning well, building up a body to suit the new expanding world. With the world of the child growing, and its experience, the way its body functions has to grow too. All very simple and quite logical with what we know about science, yet all this is ignored in favour of the theory that we are always under attack. The fight against childhood illness, like all fights against disease, can only end in defeat. To fight childhood illness is to fight development of children and as we will see later, death from childhood illness is in fact rare and if handled in a true holistic scientific manner, then illness should be seen as a rite of passage for children where they take a week off life to grow for the next stage.

Viruses

We are told viruses are in no way alive, they are "on the verge of life". Well, I suppose you could make an argument like that for just about anything. They do not do anything that constitutes life like take on food, metabolise, breathe, reproduce or create movement and energy.

So how can something that basically cannot do anything at all do all the damage it allegedly does? They claim they don't know the origin of viruses but, again, how can something that is not alive, meaning it can't reproduce, create itself? This is worse than the chicken and egg problem.

Here are some insights from qualified people.

"When a cell becomes diseased and the function of that cell begins to falter it starts to come apart at the seams. Bits of its essential structure, the DNA and RNA, may become detached as the cell itself is falling apart."

– Patrick Quanten, MD.

"We also know that viruses transfer useful genetic information from cell to cell and to other individuals in healthy cells, yet surprisingly we have never been able to show a virus infecting a host cell from the outside to the inside creating a diseased cell."

– Trevor Gunn, *The Science of Health and Healing*.

"All claims about viruses as pathogens are wrong and are based on easily recognizable, understandable and verifiable misinterpretations ... All scientists who think they are working with viruses in laboratories are actually working with typical particles of specific dying tissues or cells which were prepared in a special way. They believe that those tissues and cells are dying because they were infected by a virus. In reality, the infected cells and tissues were dying because they were starved and poisoned as a consequence of the experiments in the lab."

" ... the death of the tissue and cells takes place in the exact same manner when no "infected" genetic material is added at all. The virologists have apparently not noticed this fact. According to ... scientific logic and the rules of scientific conduct, control experiments should have been carried out. In order to confirm the newly discovered method of so-called "virus propagation" ... scientists would have had to perform additional experiments, called negative control experiments, in which they would add sterile substances ... to the cell culture."

– Dr Stefan Lanka, *The Misconception Called Virus*.

So it seems these viruses, broken down bits, waste bags of genetic material from our own diseased cells, are the result of disease and, again, not the cause. On discovering viruses in diseased patients they just replicated the Germ Theory. Yes, they are present but in no way does it show they are the cause of the disease. I have passed by fires and always see the fire brigade there but I'm pretty sure they are not arsonists. We see them after the fact and as they aren't seen unless a house is on fire it would be pure presumption to state they are causing the fires. Guilty until proven innocent is not British Law.

We don't go to the doctors when healthy so he/she wouldn't see the state of your tissues before the illness, only after, but he/she also doesn't see the process of change from healthy to diseased, this is the missing piece. It would make sense that cells are breaking down and dying every second of the day, we have natural cell death, but when cells come under too much stress excess cellular waste is seen, which in turn would mean extra viral waste bags. Now we may have what is called a viral illness. It's not cells replicating the invading virus that creates the high "viral load", it seems it's simply more cells becoming diseased and falling apart, creating more waste bags.

The exosomes (endosomes when in the cells, exosomes when excreted), that Dr Andrew Kaufman talks about could well be the viruses transferring the **"useful genetic information"** Trevor Gunn talks about and as Dr Kaufman states, they seem to be absorbing toxins and so aiding the toxic cleansing and protecting the cells. This would mean viruses and exosomes are not the same thing. Viruses are just dead waste bags of genetic material and can do nothing at all whereas exosomes actually seem to be produced by the cell with a job in mind, absorbing toxins in the cell as endosomes, and when excreted outside the cell again, absorbing toxins as exosomes though this is still a theory as Dr Kaufman has recently stated.[4]

So, what you need to ask yourself is, are viruses coming into our cells, hijacking them and getting them to reproduce the virus and leading to

---

[4] Dr. Kaufman here on exosomes:
https://www.youtube.com/watch?v=EvEeEZTD4pE

cell death? How can this happen if a virus is not only not alive but cannot even move, perceive or create its own energy, and why would something that is not alive even want to reproduce? The images of this allegedly happening are computer generated?

> **"The virus is having a field day; the desire will be to infect as many people as it can."**
>
> - UK Deputy Chief Medical Officer Jenny Harren

Where would its **"desire"** to **"infect"** people come from? Surely it takes energy to hijack another cell's energy and something that is basically dead cannot have desire. I know I don't have a medical degree but surely something is wrong in what they are trying to convince us, in that these viruses can do all the things they do yet don't seem to have any capability to do them at all.

It would seem logical, then, that when we have what is called a "viral outbreak", instead of blaming a waste bag we may need to look at other causes for mass cell breakdown, like a toxic attack or other stresses. Extra cells breaking down and dying would mean extra waste to be removed from the system. We should be looking into the environment, people's interaction with the environment – especially if there are any obvious toxins, physical or emotional, or toxins being introduced into the body in the form of vaccine programmes and medicines. Only then can we look at the individuals or communities that are being affected and try to put the pieces of the puzzle together, then all the possible factors can be seen, or there may even be one overwhelming factor in the case of a certain environmental toxin, which, again, could include the physical or emotional.

The mass media and government propaganda 24 hours a day is a very toxic attack indeed. A look at polio could give us a clue to the danger of environmental toxins. When looking into this subject and the science of virology, it all seems to be founded on a flawed theory of invading viruses and so anything built on that afterwards will automatically be wrong. Virology doesn't seem to be a science founded in proven facts at all.

The conditions after the First World War were of physical, environmental, emotional and psychological horror. Add to that experimental vaccines, over-use of Aspirin (Bayer Pharmaceutical), medical doctors always seem to think it best to do something rather than nothing, and with the belief in this invisible enemy it is hardly surprising there were mass deaths. But for that death rate to return we would need to see the return of those kind of conditions, and remember, that all happened without the extra means of creating fear we have today – modern technology and social media 24/7.

The important thing about germs and viruses is their origin. The science has told us for over a century that their origin is from within our own diseased tissue. If this is true then why are we being told to be afraid of invading bacteria and viruses from outside?

> **"If the 'germ theory of disease' were correct, there'd be no one living to believe it."**
>
> – Bartlett, Joshua Palmer, 1882-1961, father of chiropractic.

Polio

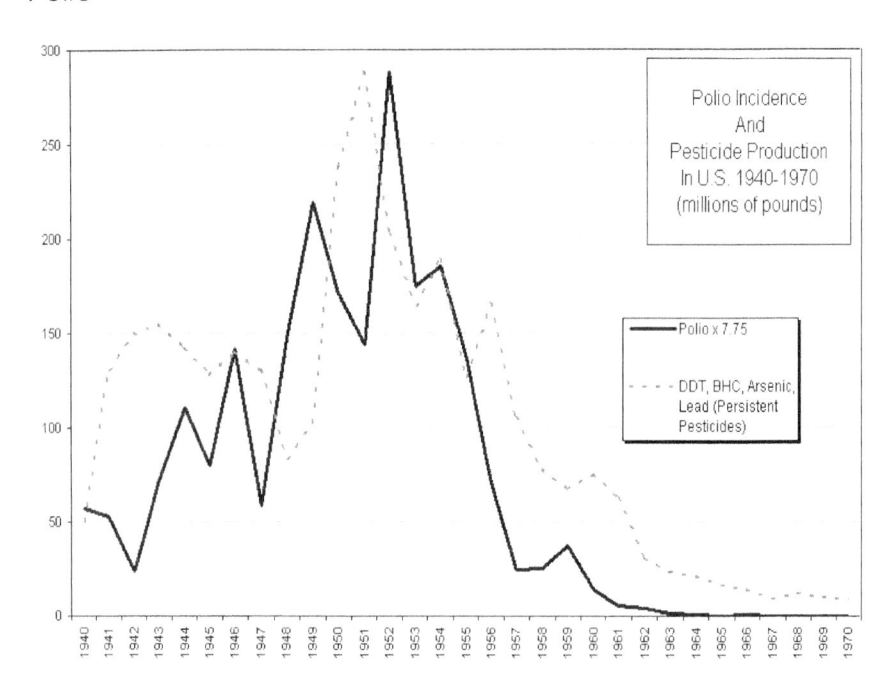

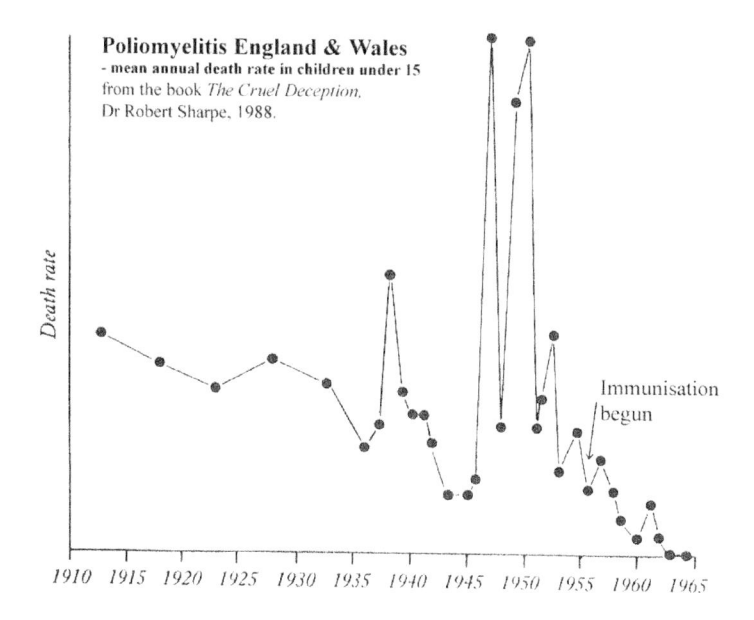

Poliomyelitis England & Wales
- mean annual death rate in children under 15
from the book *The Cruel Deception*,
Dr Robert Sharpe, 1988.

Immunisation begun

Again, after WWII, DDT pesticides were introduced and the polio death rate rises sharply.

Although this is just showing a relationship with the two, it sure is an interesting graph and does show a clear connection between polio and toxicity. Why would the medical authorities be simply ignoring data like this?

Most people think of polio as being caused by a virus. That, though, has not always been the case, indeed it was for a long time thought of as being caused by toxic poisoning. The disease has caused paralysis and death and was not known to cause epidemics until the 1900s, when major epidemics began to occur in Europe and the US. During the 1940s and 1950s, polio would paralyse or kill over half a million people worldwide every year, mainly children, giving it another name of "infant paralysis".

In 1955, a polio vaccine was developed – the Salk vaccine – and put into widespread use. Polio was itself reclassified in 1954 – what could be seen as purely coincidental, or sleight of hand British magician Paul Daniels would have been proud of. What would previously have been seen as polio could now be seen as Guillain-Barré Syndrome, transverse myelitis, coxsackie, MS, cerebral palsy.

From *The Salk 'Miracle' Myth* by Marco Cáceres, published June 2, 2015:

"In 1952, a total of 52,879 people got polio. But by 1955, the numbers had already declined by 45 percent. In 1953, 35,592 contracted polio in the US. In 1954, it was 38,476. In 1955, it was 28,985.2."

"So it is a fact of history that the numbers dropped precipitously before the Salk vaccine was widely distributed."

He then quotes Dr Bernard Greenberg, Head of the Department of Biostatistics of the University of North Carolina School of Public Health on the classification of polio:

"In order to qualify for classification as paralytic poliomyelitis, the patient had to exhibit paralytic symptoms for at least 60 days after the onset of the disease. Prior to 1954, the patient had to exhibit paralytic symptoms for only 24 hours. Laboratory confirmation and the presence of residual paralysis were not required. After 1954, residual paralysis was determined 10 to 20 days and again 50 to 70 days after the onset of the disease. This change in definition meant that in 1955 we started reporting a new disease, namely, paralytic poliomyelitis with a longer lasting paralysis."

So, it seems that polio was already in decline before the vaccine and the decline after could be a result of the reclassification alone. Ask any doctor if they are aware of this and I think the answer will be no. Control medical facts and you control medical thinking, which leads to medical treatments based on those alleged facts. Then there are the admitted cases of vaccine-induced polio which, as we will see, would not be a surprise due to the toxic nature of vaccines themselves. The WHO acknowledges circulating vaccine-derived poliovirus (cVDPV) as a reality.

Dr Stefan Lanka offered a cash prize for anyone to even prove the existence of the measles virus. After two court cases he finally won when scientists could not provide the single paper, not multiple papers, that they claimed showed the virus must exist, but the one paper that would alone prove the existence of the measles virus.

Here is an account of the trials he eventually won.

"Measles Virus put to the test. Dr. Stefan Lanka wins in court..."

The legally appointed expert Professor Podbielski in court stated, **"Thus, at this point, a publication about the existence of the measles virus that stands the test of good science has yet to be delivered."** [5]

DDT

The graphs show the connection between polio and environmental toxicity. The graphs also show us that, again, it's not just about the incoming information, in this case DDT and other toxic pesticide ingredients, but how an individual reacts to that information. Not everyone got polio but many people ate food sprayed with pesticides.

In the 1940s and 1950s, DDT was heavily used as an insecticide to attack mosquitos to combat malaria and dengue fever. In 1945, DDT was made available to farmers and for domestic use in the US but fears about its safety meant that in 1972 it was banned, except for certain public health reasons. In 2004, at the Stockholm Convention on Persistent Organic Pollutant, DDT was given a global ban with the exception of vector control, mainly for using against its old foe, the mosquito.

Though said to be moderately toxic, chronic exposure and accumulation can, according to Wikipedia, **"affect reproductive capabilities and the embryo or foetus ... Mothers with high levels of DDT circulating in their blood during pregnancy were found to be more likely to give birth to children who would go on to develop autism ... Indirect exposure of mothers through workers directly in contact with DDT is associated with an increase in spontaneous abortions"** and is **"probably carcinogenic to humans."**

So in the case of malaria and dengue have we basically just exchanged one disease for another without looking at the real cause of mosquito-borne disease? While living in the Amazon Basin in Peru for one year, I asked the medical advisor who was going into all our houses spraying them with insecticide about the dengue programme (to do it we all had to leave and they used full protection gear to go inside and spray; again, that lack of critical thinking in this world). What I was told, though, was that **"the mosquito doesn't inject the dengue virus into us but rather activates**

---

[5] https://learninggnm.com/documents/Lanka_Bardens_Trial_E.pdf

it." This from a medical professional who, with a little bit more critical thinking, would be able to see a different story.

A more complete understanding of our relationship with the mosquito is available from my good friend Dr Patrick Quanten; for me, the final piece in understanding nature and balance.

Simple question, what is the purpose of a mosquito biting an individual? [6]

So when we are seeing diseases like Ebola or HIV, or the recent Zika, we need to look at environmental toxins that may be affecting the human body, something the medical "experts" using the "best available science" either don't seem to understand or just ignore. The history of polio seems certainly connected to toxicity and a disease once thought of as a western disease could very well have been exported to the developing world, not as a virus but as toxic insecticides and other chemical poisoning, including the vaccine itself. The history of HIV, again, is a book in itself, but as we will see later the actual diagnosis of HIV is very doubtful and when seemingly healthy people are put on drugs like AZT, a known toxic cancer drug, simply because of a positive test, we have to ask the question – is the diagnosis and treatment of HIV leading to AIDS? As with "COVID", dying testing positive with HIV is not the same, especially when the test is not highlighting an actual HIV virus.

We are told that the dreaded flu virus mutates every year, therefore it is hard to prepare a vaccine for it. Again, how something that is not alive and cannot create its own energy and has no purpose does this, we won't ask, but maybe now with what we have learnt there is another option. Maybe it is not the virus itself that mutates and changes but that life itself changes. **Change is the universal constant** – so as life changes then the reasons for illness changes, ending in a different cellular breakdown, therefore different viral particles creating a different viral load.

When they claim to see viruses being replicated in a lab are they just seeing the cellular breakdown of a dying cell? This is an enormous question that needs to be answered, but by a scientific investigation in public view and with scientists with an open mind and not ones who are educated into a system with a foundation that cannot be challenged. And remembering the fact that individual susceptibly means not all are affected and that people under stress will be more susceptible, then watching the mainstream press and government daily and even hourly

---

[6] http://activehealthcare.co.uk/index.php/literature/medical/53-the-mosquito-and-i

updates is toxic in itself.

Let's face it, EVERYTHING about this life in this "system" is stress and stress is toxic.

Antivirals

What we are told about antivirals is that they reduce the ability of viruses to multiply. Seen through the eyes of germ/viral theory, it would make sense to reduce the ability of these attackers to replicate. But seeing these particles as our own cellular waste, then that would only be storing up waste and toxicity in the cells, and even though symptoms may appear to go, the cells and hence the body will be functioning at a lower level. This would be a classic example of suppression of an acute illness leading to a more chronic illness, what is called "post-viral syndrome" or as is happening now, "long COVID".

Where there is illness and drugs to be sold, there is money to be made.

> "Donald Rumsfeld has made a killing out of bird flu. The US Defence Secretary has made more than $5m (£2.9m) in capital gains from selling shares in the biotechnology firm that discovered and developed Tamiflu, the drug being bought in massive amounts by Governments to treat a possible human pandemic of the disease."
> – Independent, Sunday 12th March, 2006

> "Conflicts of interest among the UK government's covid-19 advisers"
> – BMJ, 9th December, 2020

> "By July the UK government had signed a coronavirus vaccine deal for an undisclosed sum with GlaxoSmithKline, securing 60 million doses of an untested treatment that was still being developed. In September, media outlets reported that Vallance had £600 000 (€661 000; $800 000) worth of shares in the company."

When asked on LBC radio when he discovered Sir Patrick's personal shareholding, Matt Hancock said: **"Well, I didn't know about it until I read it in the newspapers."**

BALANCE

As far as comparing going with or going against the body, I will give you a quote from Trevor Gunn in his must-read book, *The Science of Health and Healing*, when talking about possible outcomes of an acute illness.

> "**The individual resolves the illness and as a result their health is improved and they are stronger than they were before. They are less susceptible to those problems after the illness and more able to deal with them.**
>
> **The individual resolves the illness but there has been no learning as such, they are not stronger than they were before, they effectively carry on as they were before the illness, just as susceptible to succumbing to the illness as they were before.**
>
> **The illness is not resolved and as a result the health of the individual is worse than before and they descend into a lower level of chronic illness, more susceptible than before.**
>
> **The illness is not resolved and the patient is unable to react sufficiently to overcome the problem and dies.**"

Maybe we should start to see the common cold as the body telling us it's time to rest rather than something to be cured. After buying the book nearly ten years ago I can honestly say the effect the simple knowledge held within it has had on my health and that of my family, is nothing short of astounding. I used to get my regular bad cold every 18 months or so; it would start as a bad cold then turn into 2/3 days in bed. What was happening was I always tried to work through the cold stage by taking suppressive over-the-counter drugs. This would keep me going for a day or two until my body just gave up. Being self-employed, this is something I needed to avoid. In trying to keep working I only made things worse and would end up in bed for a couple of days.

On reading the book it all became very clear straight away, my body had reached its limit and waste was building up and over my balance point. I needed to rest to let the body do its job of cleansing and rebalancing. Instead of taking a day off, not eating and going to bed to rest, I carried on which in the end ended up in me losing three days' work instead of one.

Not long after reading the book I got hit by a heavy cold/flu. Determined not to do anything except stick it out, I suffered for three days. About a year later the same happened and I did the same; I think I had hot water with honey and lemon as my only intake for the first day. Since then I have only ever had one heavy cold that I could feel coming on beforehand so I finished work early, went to bed and got up midday the next day all fit and raring to go. KNOW THYSELF.

Now I remain conscious of how I am feeling and when I need to rest. By doing this I can honestly say I don't get ill, I know my limits and have taken total responsibility for my own health. As a family, since reading the book we have not needed modern medicine for maintaining health or for treating illness. When normal colds and the like come along, rest is certainly the cure. Adding fasting when a fever is present aids in detoxification, and relaxing the mind in the knowledge that the body is just doing a spring clean, all is well and it's just time to rest. There is obviously a lot more to staying in balance but best to look at the most important areas of your life, as they will have the most influence.

Clean water with life-giving energy in it, we are about 70% water ourselves after all.

Eat as much local, seasonal, natural food as you can. Food is a connection to the outside world; an exchange of information and communication. If you can't get the best food, don't worry, as Patrick Quanten says, "it's your relationship with the food that is most important." Eat when you are hungry, try not to snack, try not to eat late at night and too early in the morning. Above all, relax and enjoy your meal. The real meaning of blessing a meal is creating that energetic connection. More people now are showing how we can actually change the structure of water with our emotions. We need to literally love our food.

Get plenty of fresh air and sunshine on your skin and enjoy being in nature; it's where you are from and we need that connection.

Try to find a purpose or a passion in your life, whether in work or hobbies. Be excited to be alive.

Reduce emotional stress. Do that by reducing how important a situation is.

Reduction in the importance = reduction in stress.

Remember, life is just a game we have been created to play and healthy detachment helps to keep us sane.

Most of all, find happiness in your personal relationships and social life.

Strange these are the things that have been taken away in the name of health.

Here is Dr Patrick Quanten, from his book with Erik Bualda, *Why me? Science and spirituality as inevitable bed partners*:

What follows is all you ever need to know about the causes of disease.

- A yin disease is caused by either a larger than normal outer pressure on the individual, or a smaller than normal inner pressure coming from the individual.

- A yang is caused by either a larger than normal inner pressure coming from the individual, or a smaller than normal outer pressure on the individual. (Normal = the balance point between those two forces during the creation of the individual)

It seems life, health and disease are not as complicated as we are being led to believe. Nature seems to treat the animal kingdom well; the lion gets hurt in a hunt and goes under a bush to let the body heal, it doesn't eat and barely drinks, the body has the energy to heal and life goes on, or the wound is too severe to cope with and it dies. Now it is clear that in accident situations, modern medicine and all that goes with it can saves lives, but as soon as the emergency is over we should put our trust back in that which created us. That is nature and nature is what we are a part of and what we come out of. Nature is what created us, we should learn its laws and follow its guidelines; better to learn from the master itself than the ego-driven rebellious student.

VACCINATION ON TRIAL

Is it safe and is it effective?

> "Vaccination is a barbarous practice and one of the most fatal of all the delusions current in our time. Conscientious objectors to vaccination should stand alone, if need be, against the whole world, in defense of their conviction."
>
> – Mahatma Ghandi

> "When people ask me what are the great threats to civilisation, it's true that very unlikely things like asteroid impacts, there are those threats out there in the universe, but really I think the biggest threat to our civilisation at the moment is the disconnect in democratic societies between facts or data and the understanding of our electorates." Cox said the anti-vaccination movement "baffled" him. "In terms of vaccination, one of the great human achievements was the eradication of smallpox through a worldwide co-ordinated vaccination programme. It's probably one of the greatest achievements of modern civilisation. It killed hundreds of thousands, even millions of people throughout Europe and beyond, and it went gone. But it's clear that these childhood diseases that we've largely controlled or eradicated are going to begin rise back again if we, as a society, don't properly vaccinate our children. It's a huge risk."
>
> – Professor Brian Cox

Two very different views on vaccination.

I would be very interested in knowing if Brian Cox, the glamour boy of modern science, has ever seen the data that follows. If he did, would he change his mind? He is a scientist, after all, and it is the data that decides the truth, allegedly.

We are told:

Vaccination simulates disease

Stimulates the immune system

Creates antibodies that protect us

Saved us from infectious disease

Wiped out smallpox

Are safe and the benefits outweigh the small risk

Unvaccinated = no protection and herd immunity protects the weak

Reality

Vaccination in no way simulates disease as it has never been proven that invading microbes are the cause of infectious disease. Germ Theory is still just that, a theory. We know disease is a process that can be triggered by many factors and is not the same for every individual, and that it is a process initiated by the body to cleanse itself from a build-up of waste, toxaemia. Disease is a process and not a thing. Rather than stimulate the immune system (cleansing and rebalancing system) vaccination actually bypasses over 80% of the immune system, the digestive tract, gut flora and internal membranes, and poisons the rest with access to the internal organs, blood and brain.

Antibodies are no indication of protection; they are not specific to a particular pathogen or toxin, therefore tests can be inaccurate. It is not clear whether the test means you are infected or protected. Indeed Dr Clements of the World Health Organisation and Expanded Programme on Immunisation, in a reply to Trevor Gunn on behalf of The Informed Parent in 1995, agreed, **"there is not a precise relationship between seroresponse** (antibody production) **and protection"**.

He was replying to the fact that Trevor pointed out people with high levels of antibodies could be seen to be ill and yet people with low or no traceable antibodies could remain healthy. Also a blood antibody response could be the sign of a poor immune system as it could mean the body and especially the digestive tract is not dealing with waste and toxicity well and it is leaking deeper into the system. So by promoting the production of antibodies, it seems we are promoting the body to function in a way known to be of someone who has poor natural immune functioning.

External antibodies like those produced to protect people allergic to pollen, are not the body going wrong or an overactive immune system, surely it is the body saying that for some reason, "I don't like this, it's getting inside me and affecting me, hence I'm gonna stop it on arrival." So, blood antibodies, it seems, are produced by the body when toxicity becomes internalised. Surely it would be better to ask why that is happening. Why, though, is not a question allopathic thinking allows.

When they say a vaccine is 95% effective what they mean is in tests, mainly in the lab, a certain vaccine produced an immune response, an antibody reaction, 95% of the time, and as antibodies are not specific, how can you be sure as to which ingredient in the vaccine the body is reacting to? Remember, adjuvants are used in vaccines to actually get the immune system to respond, and again, as above, we know antibodies do not equate to protection. This statistic cannot be used to promote effectiveness in a real disease situation, it is irrelevant. Yes, the whole basis of their vaccination programme, antibodies protect us, is flawed and they know it, yet they continue with this regardless.

The graphs and letters at the end of this chapter show us vaccination never saved us from infectious disease; things like clean water and sanitation and better living conditions should take all the glory, and not Big Pharma, again supporting Soil Theory.

The smallpox death rate increased dramatically, with compulsory vaccination in the mid-1800s, then dropped off again with all infectious disease worldwide. Indeed, as Trevor Gunn mentions, symptoms of smallpox are still found in the world today under other names like monkey pox. I even remember a couple of years ago a mainstream newspaper stating a case of monkey pox in England and it being "like smallpox". Also in 1885, the people of Leicester in England came out protesting the compulsory smallpox vaccine they believed was causing damage and killing people. An estimated 100,000 people from the city and the surrounding areas went out in the streets and successfully over turned the strict compulsory vaccine law. The city introduced strict public hygiene measures and isolation of the sick, not the healthy.

With the massive fall in vaccination and the introduction of these new measures the whole world sat back and waited for a disaster to unfold. It didn't happen and in fact when other areas were still having large outbreaks and deaths with almost total vaccination rates, Leicester saw their death rate drop dramatically. Strange coincidence, Leicester was the first city in England on a regional lockdown.

This information has been kept alive in the book, *Dissolving Illusions: Disease, Vaccines, and The Forgotten History* by Suzanne Humphries MD and Roman Bystrianyk.

Here is the data deemed correct by the Dept of Health in the UK:

> "In England free smallpox vaccines were introduced in 1840 and made compulsory in 1853. Between 1857 and 1859 there were 14,244 deaths from smallpox. Between 1863 and 1865 after a population rise of 7% the death rate rose by 40.8% to 20,059. In 1867 evaders of vaccination were prosecuted. Those left unvaccinated were very few. Between 1870 and 1872 after a population rise of 9% the death rate rose by 123% to 44,840."

Did vaccines save us from smallpox? Make up your own mind.

In the 1868 book *Essay on Vaccination* by Dr Charles T. Pearce, you will see another version of the history surrounding the smallpox vaccine and its alleged success. [7]

> "Yet the Report of the Committee of the House of Commons on Jenner's discovery—on which report the money grant was made to Jenner—stated, upon the evidence given,
>
> 1st. That vaccination effectually secured the patient from small-pox.
>
> 2nd. That it never was followed by eruptions.
>
> 3rd. That it had never been known to be fatal.
>
> Every one of these assertions has been falsified. It is evident that conclusions were too hastily drawn. So fatal had been the epidemic, that a panic had seized the Parliament and the people, and then upon insufficient evidence a medical theory was established and bought most dearly by Parliament. The highest medical authorities of that day, either denounced the theory and practice of vaccination, or declined to give their assent."

---

[7] https://www.informedparent.co.uk/wp-content/uploads/2017/11/1868-The-Vaccination-An-Essay-Dr-Pearce.pdf

Sounds familiar when you look at government policies today and the lack of science backing them up.

Since the start of the Vaccine Damage Fund on 22nd March 1979, until 30th April 2017, the scheme in the UK has paid out £74,130,000. In the US the sum amounts to billions of dollars and worldwide we can only guess at a lot more. You have to be at least 60% disabled and a child/baby has to be two years or older for the parent to apply, hence any damage done at a younger age when you would think the baby's system would be more fragile and less able to deal with the toxins, does not count or at least will be very difficult to prove way after the fact. A one-off £120,000 is awarded, a pittance for a destroyed life, and this award can even affect any other benefits you may have.

With ingredients like formaldehyde, antibiotics, aluminium which is well-known to be neurotoxic, mercury-based thimerosal, animal products, human foetal cells and more, it does not take a genius to see that this can't end well. It has been well stated that the number of children actually damaged or killed by vaccines is massively underestimated due to lack of studies and nobody knows the true figure; it could be the tip of a very big iceberg.

The book, *Vaccination - 100 years of Orthodox Research Shows that Vaccines Represent a Medical Assault on the Immune System* by Viera Scheibner Ph.D. is now hard to find even on Amazon books. She showed many studies demonstrating a direct connection between vaccines and Shaken Baby Syndrome. The original link to her website is now being used by another business and her work is hard to find. What exactly is being hid?

To say vaccines are safe is simply not true. Vaccine damage payments clearly show things do go wrong and as it is the governments themselves who pay out the damages, and that itself comes from taxpayer money so we end up paying ourselves as a society for the damage done by vaccine companies. Not a bad earner if you can get it. All the profits with none of the liabilities and this policy is also going to protect the new coronavirus vaccine makers from any damages caused even though they are being pushed to rush out a vaccine in record time.

The Sunday Times, 24/10/10: **"40 deaths linked to child vaccines over seven years."**

Express, 30/12/12: **"ten deaths linked to having flu jab."** FOR 2011.

Even when proven to have been damaged, some people still don't get the payment.

"Imagine taking your healthy previously unvaccinated toddler for the MMR to see her suffer fits and never recover. Jodie is now 25 and is 80% disabled; her brain damage means that she is non verbal and her epilepsy has caused daily fits. Years after the injury the medical records revealed that actually 8 vaccines were given, 5 without consent or knowledge. The complexity, legal aid issues and the mix up with the Vaccine damage payment unit means that the family have never been compensated."[8]

If vaccines are safe why does the WHO have a vaccine safety summit?

As for the benefits, well, this letter from the WHO should explain a lot.

Trevor Gunn, a self-employed homeopath working free for The Informed Parent, a non-profit subscription magazine, asked for evidence of successful vaccine campaigns. He was sent half a dozen or so from the developing world, not the developed world, interestingly enough, and after **"diligence"** in his examination, exposing all the flaws in the reports, this was his reply.

For a full history of this letter and another great book for vaccines read *Vaccines - This Book Could Remove Your Fear of Childhood Illness* – Trevor Gunn

10 February 1998

Dear Mr Gunn

Thank you for your long letter dated 16 January. May I compliment you on your careful and expansive response to my earlier letter. I very much respect your diligence at looking at the literature and carefully considering the issues.

You ask many questions in the text of your letter which would entail a considerable amount of work on my part to answer. While of great interest to you and me, I am not sure that really benefits lay audiences. The point is that the Expanded Programme on Immunisation continues to believe in the value of child immunisations as being of overwhelming value to the human race. Until the unlikely moment we have developed perfect vaccines administered by perfect vaccinators

---

[8] https://www.arnica.org.uk/justice-for-jodie-appeal

there will remain problems from time to time. But these problems in no way mitigate against the widespread use of the vaccines. Nonetheless, national policy makers must make wise (and often difficult) decisions on what vaccines to include in the national schedule.

I do not feel that it is the right medium to embark on a scientific point-by-point defence of vaccines. My concession to this is to add that Vitamin A administration with immunisation is part of EPI's policy.

Yours sincerely

Dr C J Clements

Medical Officer, Expanded Programme on Immunisation

So the man at the head of the WHO immunisation programme and with unlimited resources didn't have the time to answer the questions raised. He said the issues raised would not **"really benefit lay audiences"**, meaning the fact that he can't stand up to the challenge of showing vaccines prevent disease is not something you and me need to know about.

He states they **"continues to believe in the value of child immunisations as being of overwhelming value to the human race"**. This confirms that vaccination benefiting mankind is a belief system and not a scientifically proven fact.

As Trevor highlighted Vitamin A deficiency as a factor in the severity of measles, they agree to **"add that Vitamin A administration with immunisation is part of EPI's policy."** So knowing this, how when a measles vaccination campaign is underway would you know if any benefit was due to the supplement or the vaccine? What do you think will take the credit?

It turns out that despite its claims, when challenged medical science cannot show one single successful vaccine campaign EVER, or simply they don't have the time and we should just take their word for it. This is where people will have to do deep study, look at their own lives and the way they function and make up their own minds about wanting to prevent a disease or stop a disease process, how much of their thinking is driven by fear, lack of knowledge or laziness, or a combination of all, and how much of that they are projecting onto other people. How much of a benefit is it to try and prevent an illness if in doing so it builds up more problems for the future? How much of a benefit is it to kill the mosquito to avoid malaria if the consequences are other diseases like polio? How much of a benefit is it to your own growth if you are always giving your decision making to "experts" in white coats?

As for unvaccinated meaning unprotected, again, we have to go back to Germ Theory and ask ourselves, protected from what? Look up the story of the "Hopewood Children" in Australia who were raised in a purely natural way without drugs or vaccines. The drop in disease due to clean water and sanitation shows clearly that "protection" is not needed and in fact just a focus on health is all that is needed to promote health in individuals and communities.

As for "herd immunity", well, that is a relatively new term and based on Germ Theory. It is based on killing the microbe and then not giving it space to survive and reproduce so that it just dies out and therefore can never come back. They say 95% "herd immunity" is needed for this to happen but as Patrick Quanten has pointed out, does the enemy suddenly give up with only 5% space left to live in? Of course not. Life always tries to continue and never gives up.

And we know that even full herd immunity doesn't seem to work.

"Whooping cough outbreak closes Texas school despite 100-percent vaccination rate: officials."

– 19th December, 2019, Fox News

If we need vaccine-induced herd immunity to protect us, how on earth are the human race and all the domestic animals now being vaccinated, still alive? Remember, modern vaccines are a relatively new invention. So if, again, the origin of germs and viruses is within our own tissues, then the idea of wiping a disease out so there is not one trace of it or even one microbe left is nonsense. As it is the conditions we live in that create disease and diseased tissues create germs from within them to clear up the waste, and viruses are part of that waste, then even if there were no smallpox viral particles left on the planet, bring back the conditions which create smallpox and it would come back. The idea of fighting disease is a war that can never be won.

In an interview I did with Dr Patrick Quanten on the history of vaccination and infections (YouTube Dr Patrick Quanten UK Column live[9]) we talk about immunity in connection to childhood illness. Meaning, if childhood

---

[9] https://www.youtube.com/watch?v=xa4dK-RV2al

illness is about development, then going through that process and allowing it to happen, and the clearing out not being suppressed and the changes being made, the child will then become "immune". Not immune from a microbial or viral attack but simply immune in the sense of not needing to go through that development process again. The body really does know what it is doing.

Herd immunity in the end is unscientific emotional blackmail and an easy way to turn people who are pro-vaccination against those who choose not to. It is claimed those who don't vaccinate put those who can't, and in some cases even those who do, at risk. Basically they are throwing their fears onto other people, a bit like the mask wearers and social distance people of today.

If vaccines protect and you are vaccinated then why attack those who don't? If vaccines are so safe then why are certain people with health issues not allowed to vaccinate?

Boosters

As Patrick points out, a vaccine is a toxic injection into the body; the body then has to prioritise the clearing-out of the toxins so any development stage (childhood illness) that the child is ready for, has to be delayed until the toxins are cleared. For allopathic doctors this means a period of vaccine protection. When the toxins are cleared out the body now has enough energy and can look to go through a development stage (childhood illness). He/she is now "susceptible" in the eyes of medical doctors but in the eyes of a holistic practitioner he/she is now ready for the next development stage. So the medical profession gives a booster, toxic injection, which then the body has to prioritise so the development stage is again put on hold. Again, in the eyes of the doctor this means a period of protection due to the vaccine's success in protecting from a virus/bacteria, simply because no illness is recorded, when in fact, according to Dr Patrick Quanten and others, the development stage is again delayed to clear out the toxins. Then when a child is older and has had all the boosters, he/she may then get an illness he/she should have had when they were five or six, and as we know, these illness seem to be more severe in older children or young adults.

Nits and worms have also been known for a long time to be connected to cleaning up the system after some kind of development which has left behind waste. The waste being pushed through the scalp would provide food for the nits and in turn they help clean up the waste.

The same could be said for worms. Where did they come from? What are they feeding on? Where and why do they seem to just go on their own? Again, why does this seem to be only in young children?

Pick your own truth. Vaccines protect from childhood illness or vaccines delay illness? Vaccines give immunity or vaccines delay immunity? Immunity is protection from a pathogen or prevention of the proliferation of certain microbes due to the terrain? The benefits are worth the risk? The choice is an individual one and not one to be chosen by society as a whole? I'm a victim or I'm in control?

Possible scenario

With the information that has been put forward now about the nature of disease and symptoms, imagine a young child having some vaccines. We know it is an injection that delivers toxins internally into the system of that child. The child then has to deal with those toxins and excrete them from the body. Maybe a day later, a week later, a month or longer the child develops a fever. The mother panics as the child seems unwell and is afraid of the high fever. In panic she gives the child Calpol which is an over-the-counter drug. The fever drops and all seems well again.

What has actually just happened? What even mainstream medicine is accepting now, is the benefits of fever in cleansing out the system.

The NICE guidelines state: **"Do not use antipyretic agents with the sole aim of reducing body temperature in children with fever."** And to put to rest the dreaded fear of febrile convulsions: **"Antipyretic agents do not prevent febrile convulsions and should not be used specifically for this purpose."**

The truth is, no one would know why a child has a fever, but if the child has had a vaccine it would be perfectly logical that in the near future a fever could be used to cleanse the toxins. The problem is allopathic thinking sees this as a side effect whereas holistic thinking sees this as an intelligent reaction. But again, using critical thinking, if the body was cleansing itself of the toxins but that cleansing was suppressed, what could be the possible consequences?

Dr Jane Donagan, in her articles in The Informed Parent, has written about many patients with meningitis who have had previous fever suppressions.[10]

Of course there may be incidents where it is not just a fever and a child is in more distress overall. Medical advice would be needed, and in certain cases it may be advised to lower fever due to other factors in that particular case but this fear of fever does seem to be damaging in the long run.

Does it seem possible to you that by stopping the process of fever, the toxins are just pushed further internally and the outcome may be meningitis? And the big question. Are our decisions driven by fear or logic?

Data not widely published

The following are graphs I copied out of the booklet "Comparing Natural Immunity with Vaccination" by Trevor Gunn and sent to the Dept. of Health through my MP. Knowing the protocol is they have to reply if it comes through your MP, I decided it was the best way to get confirmation the graphs were known to be correct. Obviously Trevor Gunn knew they were correct but I had to be sure myself and wanted proof that they knew too.

Here are copies of the graphs; sorry for the quality but it is the data that is important, and the three replies I got from the Dept. of Health. I say data not widely published but I can tell you I have not spoken to any medical professional yet, apart from my friend Patrick Quanten, who is aware of the following data.

Decide for yourself whether it is **"relevant"** or not.

Unclear dates on graphs

Diphtheria Notifications: 0-1200, Date: 1950-1988, Death Rate: 0-1000, Date: 1866-1969

Whooping Cough Notifications: 0-200,000, Date: 1950-1985

Scarlet Fever Death Rate: 0-2500, Date: 1866-1969

---

[10] http://www.jayne-donegan.co.uk/

Measles

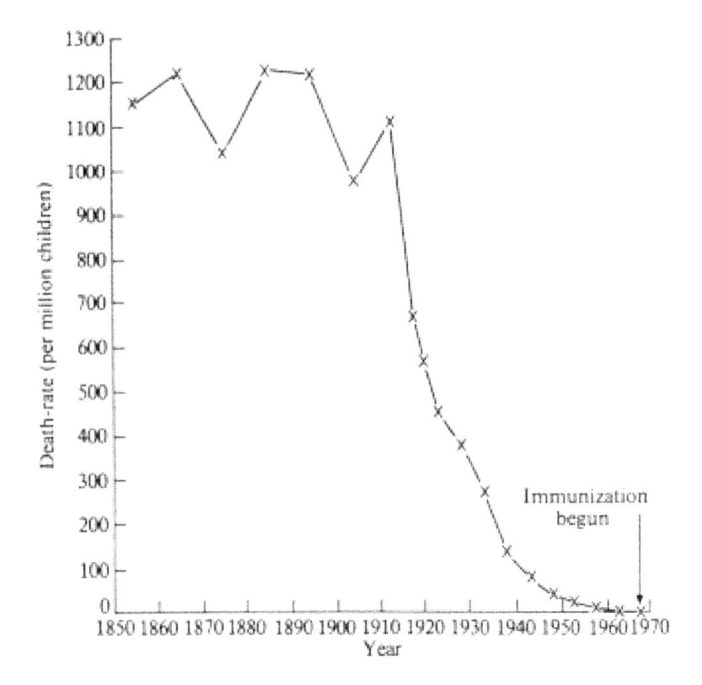

[Graph: Death-rate (per million children) vs Year, 1850–1970, showing high rates around 1100–1200 from 1850–1910, declining sharply to near zero by 1960. Arrow labelled "Immunization begun" points to around 1968.]

This is an example of a graph that doctors will **not** get in their "Green Book". It is a very powerful graph showing a very clear story. How could you imagine that this graph would not be considered **"relevant"** by the authorities? How has it even been possible to keep this graph away from public view and even doctors themselves? The fact that it has, really does show how controlled information is in this world. This graph, if released, could end the fear of measles and the risk of not vaccinating in one day. Do you think anybody would actually risk their child's health with a vaccine based on this alleged risk? With the race for the COVID vaccine do you believe the same authorities who are hiding this information will be telling you the truth about the danger of COVID-19?

It is not for me to tell anyone what conclusions to come to or who to trust but it should be very clear that we are not being told the whole truth.

Notifications of Measles to ONS
England and Wales (1940-1995)

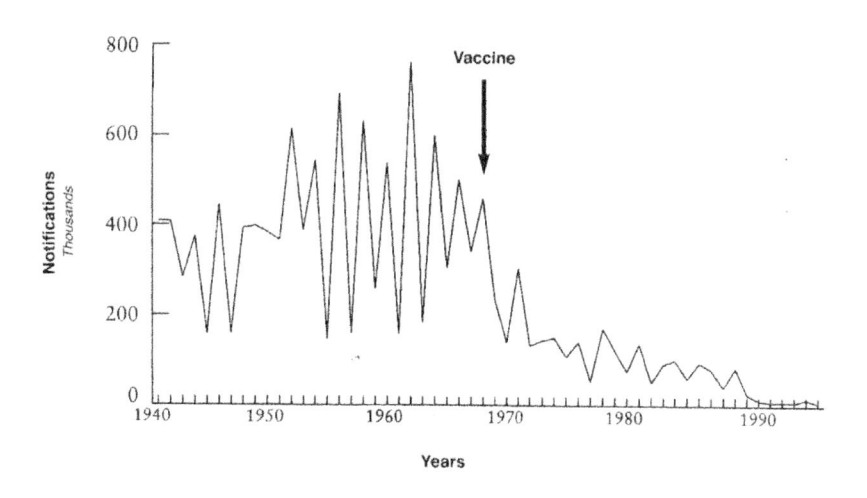

[Graph: Y-axis "Notifications (Thousands)" from 0 to 800; X-axis "Years" from 1940 to 1990. Arrow labeled "Vaccine" around 1968. Oscillating peaks between 200-800 thousand from 1940 to late 1960s, then sharp decline after vaccine introduction to low levels through the 1980s and 1990s.]

Notice the difference between when the death rate figures start and the notifications. Strange that most graphs they make public, the notifications start just before the time of the vaccine programmes. They claim they didn't have good information of notifications before that date but they did, though, have good data on deaths. Remember, as Dr Patrick Quanten mentions in the interviews, notifications are really just a guess and even alleged confirmed cases are still not really an accurate figure. People dying, though, with certain symptoms, gives us a clearer picture of the health of the population in dealing with certain illnesses. Getting an illness or testing positive is one thing and doesn't really mean anything too worrying is going on; people dying, on the other hand, would be a worry and require more investigation.

Imagine yourself as a doctor at medical school and looking at those graphs of notifications; it would surely give you the impression that vaccination is a valuable tool in preventing disease. But when you then look at the deaths the picture certainly changes and would clearly give the impression that something other than vaccines caused a massive drop in disease BEFORE vaccine programmes. Look at scarlet fever, once the biggest child killer and fell to ZERO with no vaccine programme at all.

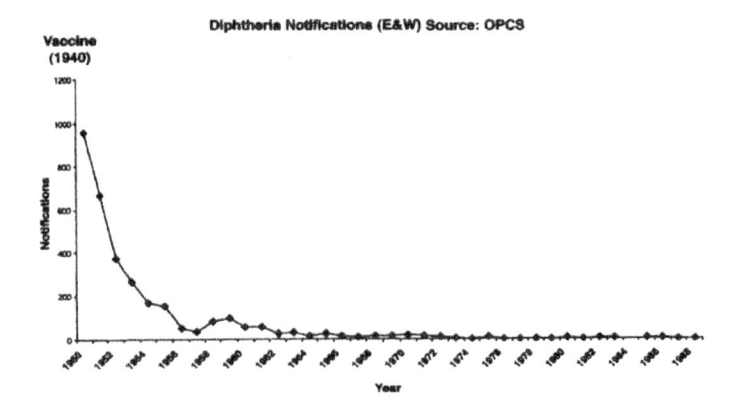

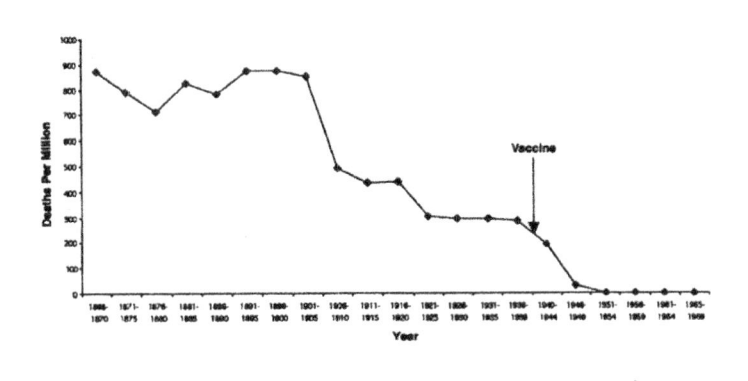

Diphtheria

Top – notifications; bottom – deaths

MEDICAL FASCISM

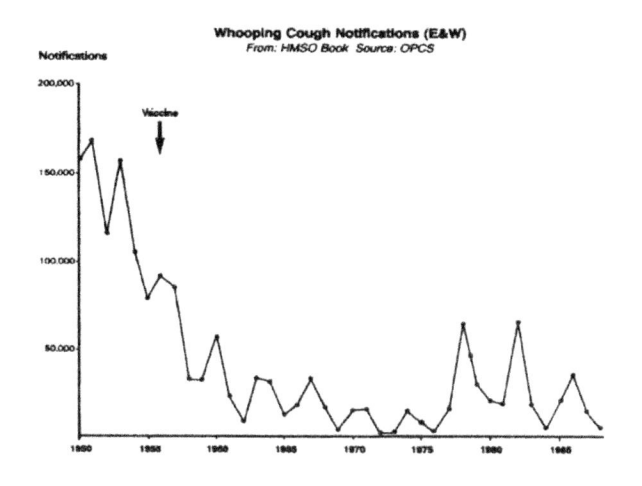

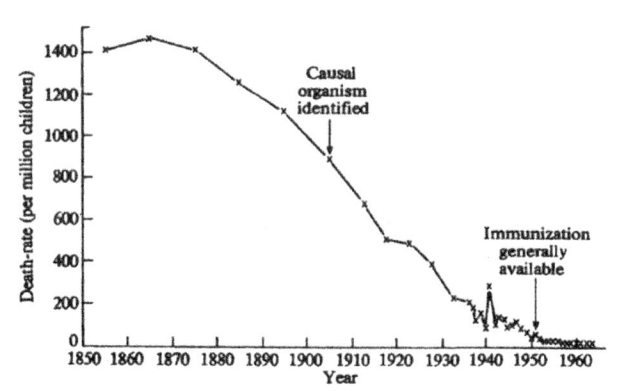

FIGURE 8.12. Whooping cough: death rates of children under 15: England and Wales.

17

Whooping cough
Top – notifications; bottom – deaths

ROB RYDER

Tetanus notification to ONS
England and Wales (1969-1995)

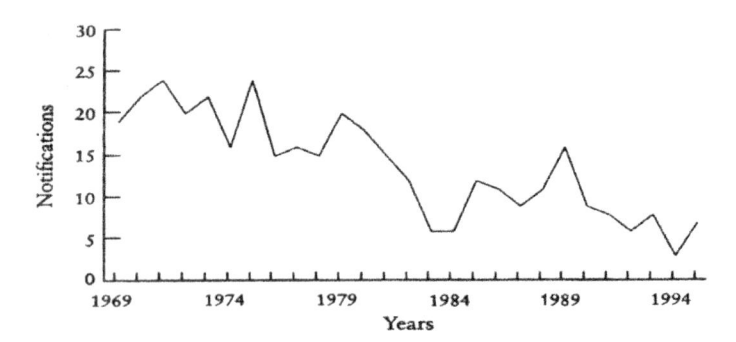

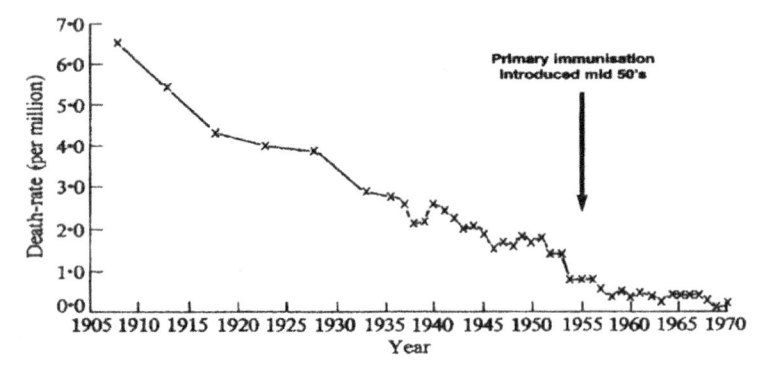

FIGURE 8.11. Tetanus: mean annual death rates: England and Wales.

18

Tetanus:
Top – notifications; bottom – deaths

Notifications of tuberculosis and deaths to ONS
England and Wales (1940-1995)

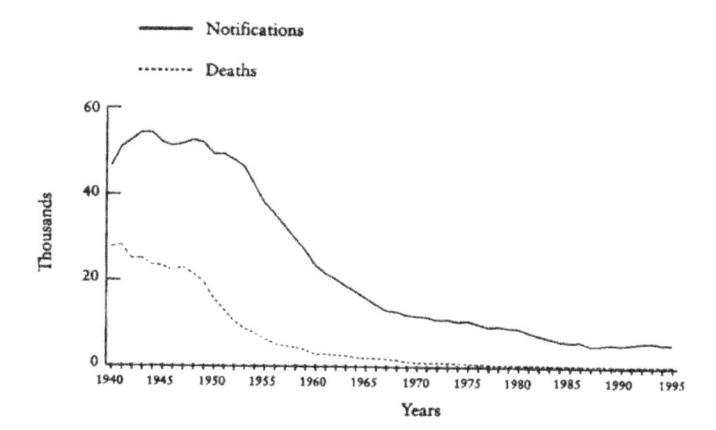

——— Notifications
·········· Deaths

Respiratory tuberculosis: mean annual death-rates E&W.

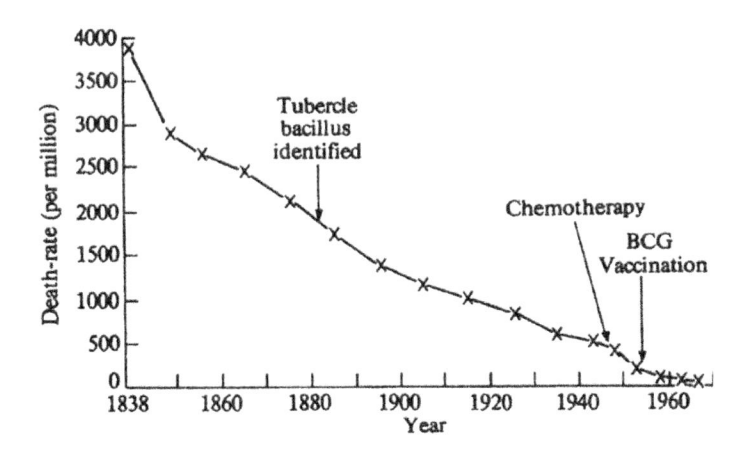

Tubercle bacillus identified

Chemotherapy

BCG Vaccination

19

Tuberculosis

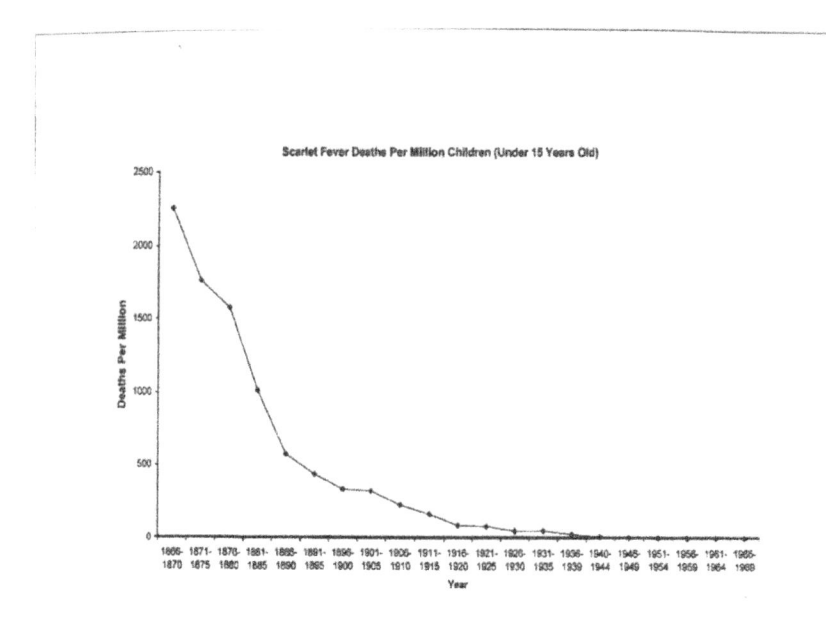

Scarlet Fever Deaths Per Million Children (Under 15 Years Old)

Above is the graph for scarlet fever, once the biggest child killer, falling to zero with no vaccine programme at all.

Fraud

> **"A false representation of a matter of facts whether by words or conduct, by false or misleading allegations, or by concealment of what should have been disclosed-that deceives and is intended to deceive another so that the individual will act upon it to her or his legal injury."**

Below are the three letters I received from Jane Ellison MP, the Parliamentary Undersecretary of State for Public Health at the time, regarding my questions about vaccines, cancer and fluoride. Apologies, but I wanted to use the original copies.

MEDICAL FASCISM

Department of Health

Your Ref: 14/18.1/ag/ew

PO00000841071

Andrew George MP
Trewella
18 Mennaye Road
Penzance TR18 4NG

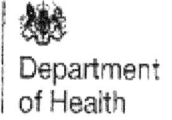

From Jane Ellison MP
Parliamentary Under Secretary of State for Public Health

Richmond House
79 Whitehall
London
SW1A 2NS

Tel: 020 7210 4650

0 6 MAR 2014

Dear Andrew

Thank you for your letter of 6 February on behalf of your constituent about the publication *Comparing Natural Immunity with Vaccination* by Trevor Gunn.

Public Health England (PHE), the national organisation for the improvement of public health outcomes, has provided the following information.

As Mr Ryder may be aware, the Government is advised on all immunisation matters by the Joint Committee on Vaccination and Immunisation (JCVI), which is an independent Departmental Expert Committee and a statutory body. In providing advice and making recommendations, it considers all currently available relevant evidence, including both published and unpublished information from a variety of sources. These sources include, but are not limited to, publications by scientists in peer-reviewed journals, opinion of experts in the field and information provided by vaccine manufacturers. Data from the Office for National Statistics, some of which are unpublished, may also be reviewed. The recommendations of the JCVI are translated into guidelines for best practice which are published in the 'Green Book' *Immunisation against Infectious disease*, a PHE publication.

Comparing Natural Immunity with Vaccination is the opinion of one individual and is not a peer-reviewed publication. It would not be considered as a reliable source of information for consideration by the JCVI. The JCVI takes into account reliable data on disease and death as a result of vaccine-preventable infectious diseases. These data are provided by surveillance schemes such as those run by PHE. More information on these surveillance schemes and links to reports and data can be found on the website www.hpa.org.uk by selecting 'topics A-Z' and then 'vaccinations'.

Such data are considered when JCVI decisions are made and used to develop information which appears in the Green Book.

Mr Gunn criticises a solely orthodox medical approach to health and illness and suggests that there are other ways in which serious disease can be avoided. Unfortunately, the data in the publication, which   included in his letter, only show death rates in England and Wales. By failing to consider the effects of vaccination on the impact of serious disease (as well as death), these graphs do not give an accurate picture of the impact of immunisation on public health.

The very large decreases in death rates in England and Wales that are shown in the figures since the late 1800s may be due to a variety of factors, including improved sanitation and a better understanding of the ways in which transmission of infectious diseases can be prevented. There is no evidence to suggest that the transient increase in death rates due to smallpox in the 1870s was causally related to the introduction of the vaccine. The introduction of the smallpox vaccine had a dramatic effect on the incidence of disease and death worldwide and resulted in the World Health Organization announcing in 1980 that smallpox had officially been eradicated.

With regard to issues of consent, immunisation in the United Kingdom is based on informed consent. Consent must be obtained before starting any treatment or physical investigation or before providing personal care for a patient. This includes the administration of all vaccines.

The NHS Choices website states that *for consent to be valid, it must be voluntary and informed, and the person consenting must have the capacity to make the decision*" and that *the person must be given full information about what the treatment involves, including the benefits and risks, whether there are reasonable alternative treatments, and what will happen if treatment does not go ahead.*

PHE provides a range of leaflets, newsletters and other sources of information which are freely available and which enable people to make informed decisions about accepting medical treatment, including vaccination. In addition, healthcare workers discuss the possible implications of treatment (both positive and negative) with individuals prior to that treatment being given.

Finally, the JCVI, PHE and the Department of Health only consider issues which affect human, not animal, health and so I am unable to comment on any possible relationship between immunisation programmes in people and vaccination of badgers as a means of controlling bovine TB. This issue is one for the Department for Environment, Food and Rural Affairs.   may therefore wish to contact that Department for more information. The contact details are:

**Department
of Health**

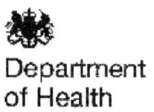

Department for Environment, Food and Rural Affairs
Nobel House
17 Smith Square
London SW1P 3JR

I hope this reply is helpful.

*Kind regards
Jane*

JANE ELLISON

Notes on letter

The government is advised by the JCVI in **"providing advice and making recommendations"** and **"considers all currently available relevant evidence"**, which is **"translated into guidelines for best practice which are published in the Green Book immunisation against infectious disease"**.

So to be clear, the JCVI does not think it is **"relevant"** to publish to doctors the massive fall in death rate from infectious disease, total fall in case of scarlet fever, happening BEFORE vaccine programmes. They say that the book which I used to quote the data, *Comparing Natural Immunity with Vaccination* by Trevor Gunn, would **"not be considered a reliable source of information for consideration by the JCVI"**. But the source of the information is the ONS, a government organisation which takes data from the medical profession. So are they saying their own data is not reliable?

They also claim the JCVI would not consider it a reliable source of information. So the question is, have the JCVI even seen this data? Is it being deliberately withheld? Have they seen it but decided themselves it is not **"relevant"**? The answer to these questions I have yet to investigate.

Jane Ellison admits the **"very large decreases in death rate"** were due to **"a variety of factors including improved sanitation"**. And on seeing the smallpox data shown earlier with the rise with compulsory vaccines, she admitted there was a **"transient increase in death rate due to smallpox"** but it was not **"causally related to the introduction of the vaccine"**. So without any investigation it was just a coincidence. She stated, **"the introduction of the smallpox vaccine had a dramatic effect on the incidence of the disease and death worldwide"**. In this she is right but the dramatic effect was the dramatic rise in the death rate.

I have only used the England and Wales figures as those are the ones I can confirm with our own Dept. of Health but by reading the book *Dissolving Illusions: Disease, Vaccines, and The Forgotten History* by Suzanne Humphries MD and Roman Bystrianyk, you will be able to see other world figures showing the same story with a rise in death from smallpox with the vaccine.

Reading the book *Nature Cure* by Henry Lindllar you will see another version of the smallpox history and view of the hero Edward Jenner, and that it wasn't true that those milk maids who had cowpox were immune to smallpox; in fact it is another story similar to that other hero Lous Pasteur, in that a particular viewpoint was taken on board as truth despite having very little scientific basis and many scientists in their time not agreeing with their conclusions.

Surely to use the term **"vaccine preventable infectious disease"** you would need to show they actually prevent it in the first place. The **"law of consent"** is mentioned so she must be fully aware of what it entails.

Law of Consent

Consent from a patient is needed regardless of the procedure, whether it's a physical examination, organ donation or something else.

Defining consent

> **For consent to be valid, it must be voluntary and informed, and the person consenting must have the capacity to make the decision.**
>
> **Voluntary – the decision to either consent or not to consent to treatment must be made by the person, and must not be influenced by pressure from medical staff, friends or family.**
>
> **Informed – the person must be given all of the information about what the treatment involves, including the benefits and risks, whether there are reasonable alternative treatments, and what will happen if treatment does not go ahead.**
>
> **Capacity – the person must be capable of giving consent, which means they understand the information given to them and can use it to make an informed decision.**

When consent is not needed is a risk to public health as a result of rabies, cholera or T.B. (Seems COVID-19 has just been added to that list.)

In your opinion are we being **"informed"**? I personally don't think so, and after years of research I am actually shocked at how little doctors know about vaccines and their history.

ROB RYDER

Department of Health

Your ref: 14/18.1/ag/jr

PO00000880159

Andrew George MP
Trewella
18 Mennaye Road
Penzance TR18 4NG

— 8 SEP 2014

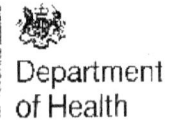

From Jane Ellison MP
Parliamentary Under Secretary of State for Public Health

Richmond House
79 Whitehall
London
SW1A 2NS

Tel: 020 7210 4850

0 5 SEP 2014

Dear Andrew

Thank you for your letter of 5 August on behalf of your constituent Mr Robert Ryder of ⸻ about water fluoridation.

Tooth decay remains a public health problem with wide inequalities between communities. It is also one of the most common reasons for children to be admitted to hospital.

The research evidence suggests that fluoridating water is the most effective step we can take to reduce tooth decay generally at a population level, both among children and adults. The ideal combination for good dental health is likely to involve drinking fluoridated water, professionally delivered dental care and helping people adopt healthy lifestyles.

Most water supplies contain some natural fluoride content and around half a million people in the UK receive naturally fluoridated water at levels close to those achieved by fluoridation schemes. Over five million people in England are served by water supplies where the level of fluoride has been adjusted to the recommended level of one part per million. There are extensive water fluoridation schemes in the USA serving over 200 million people, and similar schemes operate in a number of other countries, such as Australia. The chemicals used by water companies in England to adjust levels of fluoride are procured specifically for this purpose and are highly regulated.

As Mr Ryder is aware, water fluoridation has been extensively studied and reviewed over the last 50 years. In the UK, the most recent review was undertaken by the NHS Centre for Reviews and Dissemination based at the University of York and published in 2000. In 2002, the Medical Research Council reported to the

Department of Health its advice on future research priorities. The US National Research Council reported in 2006 and the Australian National Health and Medical Research Council reported in 2007. The evidence from these reports is that community water fluoridation schemes are effective in reducing tooth decay levels and there is no evidence that these schemes are a cause of general ill health.

The fluoride chemicals used to fluoridate drinking water are hydrofluorosilicic acid, sodium fluorosilicate, and sodium fluoride. Water companies are only permitted to use specified fluoridation chemicals in accordance with European standards. These standards specify purity levels and producers are not permitted to sell chemicals unless these purity criteria are met.

Under the Health and Social Care Act 2012, a new approval process was introduced on the way that the NHS and public health service introduce fluoridation schemes. The Act transfers responsibility for consultations on proposals for new fluoridation schemes to local authorities. Not only will this increase democratic accountability but also, in preparing new regulations on the conduct of consultations, ministers will be looking to ensure that fuller account of the views of the people that would be affected is taken in decisions on fluoridation.

The Government is resolved that decisions on any new schemes are taken locally after wide ranging consultation. I would like to assure Mr Ryder that no scheme should go ahead unless there was clear local support, and both opponents and supporters of fluoridation have been given a platform to discuss their views.

I also note Mr Ryder's concerns about immunisation. Research from around the world shows that immunisation is the safest and most effective way to protect children against infectious diseases that can cause serious long-term ill-health, including mental and/or physical disability, and premature death. The UK's childhood immunisation programme has resulted in a very low incidence of childhood infectious diseases. For example, diphtheria, polio and neonatal tetanus no longer occur in UK children.

The vaccinations included in the NHS routine childhood immunisation schedule have been recommended by experts after consideration of a wide range of evidence including evidence about efficacy and safety. The vaccines have undergone rigorous testing with large numbers of people before being licensed, and their safety is continuously monitored to discover and assess any rare side-effects. These recommended vaccines are among the safest medicines available.

Vaccine safety is of paramount importance and, as with all vaccines and medicines, the Medicines and Healthcare products Regulatory Agency and the Government's

Department of Health

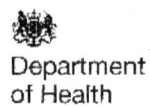

independent expert advisory Commission on Human Medicines keeps the safety of vaccines under close and continual review.

I hope this reply is helpful.

Kind regards
Jane

JANE ELLISON

Apologies again for the quality of the copies but as you can see, these are the original letters.

> **"the research evidence suggests that fluoridating water is the most effective step we can take to reduce tooth decay."**

Watch YouTube – "The Fluoride Deception"

Yes, she is right, most waters supplies contain natural fluoride but to **"adjust"** the levels they use **"chemicals" a**nd not natural fluoride. The NHS website on fluoride again mentions natural fluoride but omits to mention these other **"chemicals"** that are used to fluoridate water supplies and toothpaste. They do mention, **"There have been some concerns that fluoride may be linked to a variety of health conditions. Reviews of the risks have so far found no convincing evidence to support these concerns."** But do admit to **"a condition called dental fluorosis"**. Whatever the health risks may or may not be, the clear fact is this is at least not fulfilling the **"law of consent"** again and is at least misleading and at worst fraud that is causing damage. Again, if we had open investigations and open, honest science with all the facts on display we would be able to come to a better conclusion.

She again mentions vaccines are a **"safe and most effective way to protect children against infectious diseases"** when knowing that vaccine damage is real and things like clean water and sanitation lead to the massive drop in deaths before vaccines. And insists again it is the vaccine programmes that have caused the low incidence of disease. There is a term called cognitive dissonance when someone can hold two opposing views at one time. Either Jane Ellison is suffering from cognitive dissonance, or speaking some kind of "double speak", or is just repeating information she is getting off a screen without even looking at it herself. Whatever her own personal truth, one thing is for sure that none of the official truth makes any sense at all.

As she states, the chemicals used are: **hydrofluorosilicic acid, sodium fluorosilicate, sodium fluoride**.

Here is one example of the dangers from Wikipedia:

> **"Sodium fluoride is classed as toxic by both inhalation (of dusts or aerosols) and ingestion."**

Department of Health

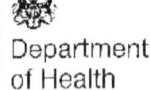

Your Ref: 14/18.1/ag/ew

PO00000865738

Andrew George MP
Trewella
18 Mennaye Road
Penzance TR18 4NG

- 7 JUL 2014

From Jane Ellison MP
Parliamentary Under Secretary of State for Public Health

Richmond House
79 Whitehall
London
SW1A 2NS

Tel: 020 7210 4850

0 3 JUL 2014

Dear Andrew

Thank you for your letter of 4 June on behalf of your constituent Mr Robert Ryder of ~~[redacted]~~ about immunisation.

Research from around the world shows that immunisation is the safest way to protect a child's health. The vaccinations included in the NHS routine childhood immunisation schedule have been recommended by experts, after consideration of a wide range of evidence, including evidence about efficacy and adverse reactions. The vaccines have undergone rigorous testing with large numbers of people before being licensed and their safety is continuously monitored to discover and assess any rare side effects. These recommended vaccines are among the safest medicines.

Immunisation protects children against diseases which, even today in developed countries, can cause serious long-term ill-health, including mental and/or physical disability, and even kill. The childhood immunisation programme in the UK has resulted in the incidence of childhood diseases being at very low levels.

In the UK, these diseases are kept at bay by high immunisation rates. Around the world, more than 15 million people a year die from infectious diseases. More than half of these are children under the age of five. Most of these deaths could be prevented by immunisation. As more people travel abroad and more people come to visit this country, there is a risk that they will bring these diseases into the UK. The diseases may spread to people who have not been immunised.

As set out in my previous reply (our ref: PO00000841071), the Government is advised on all immunisation matters by the Joint Committee on Vaccination and Immunisation (JCVI), and Mr Ryder, or you on his behalf, may therefore wish to contact it directly.

With regard to Mr Ryder's concerns about cancer, the Department of Health is fully committed to clinical and applied research into treatment and cures for cancer. The Department's National Institute for Health Research (NIHR) welcomes funding applications for research into any aspect of human health, including cancer. These applications are subject to peer review and judged in open competition, with awards being made on the basis of the scientific quality of the proposals made. The NIHR spends around £100million annually on cancer research.

In August 2011, the Department of Health announced the UK's largest ever investment, £800million, in 'early stage' health research that will fund advances in diagnosis, prevention and treatment, benefiting patients with diseases including cancer, diabetes and heart disease. Of the £800million, £61.5million is for the NIHR biomedical research unit in cancer, a partnership between the Royal Marsden Hospital and the Institute of Cancer Research.

I hope this reply is helpful.

Kind regards
Jane

JANE ELLISON

After just repeating the theme about vaccines, in the final letter Jane Ellison also addresses my concerns over cancer. It seems, as usual, the same reply of just totally ignoring any possible investments into natural therapies and as on other NHS pages, they just attack **"alternative"** therapies or say there is no evidence. Well, if you don't look, you won't find. The truth is, cancer is a multi-billion-pound business and there are too many invested interests to risk anyone finding a cure, especially if that cure lay within the body of the individual. Like all diseases, cancer is a process and not a thing and by understanding how it advances we may come to understand how to reverse it. To do that, though, would take holistic thinking and a desire to give health and not make profit.

One thing for sure from looking at the data and seeing the letters, is that we are not being told the truth and in that case, how can the **"law of consent"** be applied?

Looking at the "Coronavirus Act 2020" you can see a clear attack on the law of consent. Even for a physical examination consent is needed but it seems the Coronavirus Act has taken that protection away completely, as we will see further on.

So where do we now stand exactly? Is a law that has been passed by a process and put in place to protect our natural rights under common law now not valid because of an alleged state of emergency? It does seem now that the word of one man, Boris Johnson, can overpower the laws of a nation; this is clearly a dictator's actions. So looking at the law, please now examine your experience when being asked to vaccinate or for that matter take any medical treatment or drug. Clearly by not giving us, or even doctors in their Green Book, all the evidence, then it is impossible for doctors to give out full information on the benefits of vaccines if they are given such a one-sided view. I would also surely doubt they are aware of the massive vaccine damage pay-outs and I have never known them to give alternatives.

Dr Jane Donegan was charged with serious professional misconduct after being accused by senior judge of using **"junk science"** after she wrote two reports for a case heard in 2002 in the family division of the High Court, relating to two families who were unconnected but whose cases became linked in the courts. Although the courts lodged no complaint, the GMC began an investigation and announced that Dr Donegan would face a charge of serious professional misconduct. In 2007 after a three-week hearing in Manchester, the GMC panel concluded that all of the substantive charges against Dr Donegan were unproved except for the charge of quoting selectively from research. The panel declared, however, that "**it is normal practice in the preparation of reports to quote selectively from references, which indeed you did.**"

Sheila Hewitt, who chaired the panel, told Dr Donegan: "**The panel were sure that at no stage did you allow any views that you held to overrule your duty to the court and the litigants. You demonstrated to the panel that your report did not derive from your deeply held views, and your evidence supported this.**"

What was Dr Donegan's crime?

She backed the mothers' stance in opposing the MMR and other childhood immunisations.

Jane, along with Patrick Quanten, writes for The Informed Parent.[11]

The Informed Parent was founded by Magda Talylor who has done nearly 29 years of amazing research into the history of vaccines and infectious disease. Her stunning interview on the Jason Liosatos Show "Outside the Box" on YouTube – "**Vaccination Facts, History Lesson and Interview with Magda Taylor**" – where she starts from just before the famous Jenner, smallpox period is a must watch. If you have got this far and you still have an open mind then watching this interview is a must for a very detailed look at how information was continually ignored by areas of the scientific community and politicians who had taken hold of a theory and decided to push it forward as scientific truth, no matter what evidence from other scientists and medical doctors. Yes, even in those times the politicians were claiming to be using the "best available science" and as you will see, history does seem to be repeating itself again in more ways than one.

The Informed Parent is one of few organisations I support and I can recommend subscribing and helping Magda in her incredible work.

---

[11] https://www.informedparent.co.uk/

THE HISTORY OF MODERN MEDICINE

"To find health should be the object of the doctor. Anyone can find disease."

– Andrew Taylor Still, 1828-1917. Father of osteopathy.

Modern medicine, allopathic medicine, means to oppose. Oppose what the body is doing. This is the only accepted scientific method, thinking and truth but it wasn't always like this. In fact, as Patrick Quanten points out in my interview with him, it is actually modern medicine which is the alternative. Traditional means what is longstanding and as far as history is concerned modern medicine is a newcomer.[12]

Around the time of modern medicine getting started and changing the way we see and therefore treat disease, a peasant farmer, in Gräfenberg, Austria, lay the foundations of what became known as Nature Cure. Vincenz Priessnitz, 1799-1851. Born into a farmer's family he grew up observing nature and especially what animals did when ill or suffering wounds. Copying their methods, he became very well versed in what would become to be known as hydrotherapy, using water to heal, with the addition of other natural therapies such as vegetarian food, air, sunlight, exercise, rest, water, fasting and traditional medicine (remember, traditional means longstanding). His reputation grew and in 1822 he extended his father's home to build a healing spa for the incoming patients.

His therapies, which did not use modern drugs or even herbal remedies, were focused on removing waste matter and foreign matter from the body, whose build-up became known as the cause of disease in "toxaemia". Waste is a matter of life; we take in food, air and liquids and in the modern world toxins in the diet and environment. The idea is the body removes the waste so it remains at a balanced level which does not disturb the functioning of the body. Many things like poor diet, overeating, lack of exercise, a toxic environment and poor organ function that may

---

[12] YouTube – "Patrick Quanten: Modern Medicine - truth lies in the history" https://www.youtube.com/watch?v=HmW_6QKqvq0

be due to stress, can build up waste.

In recent times, through "German New Medicine" and other practices, we now know how the emotions can affect the body, certain emotions affecting certain parts of the body and therefore how it functions. When waste builds up and goes beyond your balance point then an extra effort is needed by the body to remove the excess waste and restore balance; this was the principle behind his healing and something only the body itself could do. We could help it by removing stresses and partaking in certain natural therapies but the healing was up to the body.

The success of his natural nontoxic methods saw him even treating royalty and in 1846, Priessnitz was awarded a medal by the Emperor. The world, though, would soon forget the peasant farmer from Austria and was given a path instead that would see modern medicine not just creating a near monopoly on health and disease but even attacking the more traditional practitioners as "Quacks".

Toxic takeover

The American Medical Association – AMA – founded in 1847 and incorporated in 1897, is the largest association of physicians – both MDs and DOs – and medical students in the United States. Their mission was to **"to promote the art and science of medicine and the betterment of public health."** Its founder, Nathan Smith Davis, also founded the Journal of the American Medical Association in 1883 and was behind pushing laws for compulsory smallpox vaccines in 1889.

In 1904 the AMA created the Council on Medical Education (CME) with the aim of restructuring the American medical education. In 1908 the CME contacted the Carnegie Foundation for the Advancement of Teaching to survey the American medical education. Abraham Flexner was chosen to conduct the survey although he was neither a physician, scientist nor medical educator. After visiting 155 of the medical schools in America, all very diverse in their thinking, he came back using the John Hopkins School of Medicine as his ideal in 1910 and with these recommendations:

Reduce the number of medical schools (from 155 to 31) and poorly trained physicians.

Increase the prerequisites to enter medical training.

Train physicians to practice in a scientific manner and engage medical faculty in research.

Give medical schools control of clinical instruction in hospitals.

Strengthen state regulation of medical licensure.

This report was then pushed through the colleges and hospitals with an initial donation of $100 from John D. Rockefeller; many hundreds of millions followed. The report basically regulated all of medical thinking and training with oversight given to the AMA and made allopathic thinking and Germ Theory unchallenged as the only acceptable scientific way to deal with illness and disease. From this day on, disease became a massive business, one that the Rockefeller Foundation invested in – yes, invested in, and not donated. We then saw an onslaught against any other health practices such as homeopathy, chiropractic, osteopathy, naturopathy and more and also an attack on anyone against the use of vaccines to prevent disease; the term "quackery" had been invented.

I find it also interesting that a similar attack on marijuana happened in the US around the same time. A plant well known for its many uses and medicinal qualities, after years of attacks in regulating it, the 1937 Marijuana Tax Act was the beginning of the end for this highly useful bit of nature. It was then classified as a narcotic drug in the US, bringing an end to the easy access of this wonder of nature. Strangely, again, this plant was a huge competitor to the now-Rockefeller-backed big pharma and even his oil business. Maybe the competition was just pushed out of the way?

The later establishment of the WHO was, again, centred on allopathic thinking and Germ Theory, hence mass promotion of vaccines and claims they wiped out smallpox with vaccines. But to understand the Flexner Report is to understand the position we find ourselves in today and how the WHO and the Rockefeller-backed science took hold of the world. The same family who were well known to use homeopathy.

This is the same Rockefeller Foundation that in 1939 formed an alliance with the German chemical company I.G. Farben. I.G. Farben was once the largest chemical and pharmaceutical company in the world and owned the Monowitz concentration camp, which was a subcamp of the main Auschwitz concentration camp and used to produce chemicals for I.G. Farben with the slave labour provided by the Nazis from the main concentration camp at a cheap rate. Employees of the Bayer group at I.G. Farben conducted medical experiments on concentration camp inmates and the company was a massive powerful ally and funder of the Nazis.

After the war I.G. Farben was broken up into its original companies and one of them, Bayer, in 2016 bought the infamous Monsanto Company for $66 billion and took control of GMO seeds. Bayer was also the creators of aspirin before they merged into I.G. Farben, an interesting fact we went into when looking at treatments of the great Spanish Flu.

At the Nuremberg trials directors of I.G. Farben were put on trial for war crimes and thirteen were found guilty. Also research "Operation Paperclip" for information on how Nazi scientists were brought to the west after the war ended.

There is a massive story surrounding the Nazis and private companies that could entail a book by itself but the point I want to make is that the people who run and control medical thinking, allegedly to help human suffering, took part in some of the worst atrocities against human beings.

This modern way of looking at things goes against the well-established sciences going back thousands of years from Ayurveda and later Chinese medicine. These sciences took into account the whole human being and not just the physical symptom; life was about energy and an expression of energy, something we knew from before the time of Einstein, yet have continued to ignore in medical science to this day and to the detriment of human health. Until the true nature of what we are, energy and emotional, is incorporated into health and our understanding of disease, I'm afraid human health will only deteriorate as big pharma profits rise.

In the UK: The Cancer Act 1939

> **"No person shall take part in the publication of any advertisement**
>
> **A: containing an offer to treat any person for cancer or to prescribe any remedy therefor, or to give any advice in connection with the treatment thereof."**

Here we now see the correct medical science and organisations using government to take total control of the treatment of disease, even criminalising anyone claiming to treat or cure cancer without the correct method. Only a medical doctor can now treat cancer and the main three methods they have used for decades is chemotherapy, radiotherapy and surgery, and yet cases rise and the cost of treating continues to go into the billions. Welcome to the cancer business.

As for alternatives, just look at what happened to the Gerson Institute in the US, banned despite having masses of documented cases of "curing" cancer with natural detoxification therapies with natural juices and supplements. They were kicked out into Mexico for their crimes. This attack continues today in the UK with David Noakes being imprisoned for four charges relating to the manufacture, sale and supply of an unlicensed medicine, GcMAF. Though GcMAF is not a pharmaceutical drug and derived from a naturally occurring human protein, the medical establishment, the government and the courts all waged war against this man who similar to the "Gerson Therapy", had many testimonials to the effectiveness of treating cancer without the awful and sometimes deadly side effects of modern doctor-prescribed treatments. The evidence seemed clear, it was safe and could actually be a major breakthrough in treating cancer, but that did not matter at all, he wasn't a doctor and he didn't follow protocol therefore he is a criminal. Not that he had actually harmed anyone, in fact the opposite, but in the eyes of the establishment he was a danger to society.[13]

Toxic Psychiatry

There is a stunning book, *Toxic Psychiatry* by Peter R Breggin MD. I recommend reading it to get an insight into the massive damage modern medical thinking, doctors and drug companies have done to humanity over the last century. Psychiatry is really just an extension of this system concentrating on what is known as "mental illness". Psychiatrists are in fact medical doctors so we see straight away how they are trained in medical school, this time seeing mental illness or psychiatric problems as things going wrong and again, based on materialism.

A look into the history and the same names come up again.

Ernest Rudin, 1874-1922, worked under Emil Kraepelin who was known as the founder of modern scientific psychiatry, psychopharmacology and

---

[13] For more information on David Noakes go to www.ukcolumn.org

psychiatric genetics. Rudin was a Swiss-born German psychiatrist, geneticist, eugenicist and Nazi. He has been credited as a pioneer of psychiatric inheritance studies and in 1932 he became President of the International Federation of Eugenics Organizations.

Rüdin joined the Nazi Party in 1937 and in 1939, he was awarded a 'Goethe medal for art and science' handed to him personally by Hitler, who honoured him as the 'pioneer of the racial-hygienic measures of the Third Reich'. In 1944 he received a bronze Nazi eagle medal, with Hitler calling him the 'pathfinder in the field of hereditary hygiene'. He also held the post of professor of psychiatry at the Kaiser Wilhelm Institute in Munich which later inspired and conducted Eugenics experiments in the Third Reich, the same institute that when having financial problems in the early 1930s, was bailed out by that family again, the Rockefeller Foundation.

He was also a visitor in America with the support of that other great family; yes, you guessed it, the Carnegie Foundation. As Breggin states in his book **"it was Rudin who influenced Hitler, not Hitler who influenced Rudin"**.

During the late 1920s, the Rockefeller Foundation created the Medical Sciences Division which was known for making large contributions to research across several fields of psychiatry. The horrific legacy of this is well-documented in *Toxic Psychiatry*. It was an era with the Rockefeller Foundation giving massive donations to the fields of psychiatry, social sciences and genetics and continued funding Nazi racial studies even after it was clear that this research was being used to rationalise the demonising of Jews and other groups. They continued to fund Nazi racial science studies at the Kaiser Wilhelm Institute of Anthropology, Human Heredity, and Eugenics up until 1939, four years after the 1935 Nuremberg Laws which were a racist assault on all non-Germans by the Nazi Party.

If we think of what is happening to our children in schools today with all the "safety" rules to follow, think of what Peter Breggin said in chapter 12 of his book, entitled: **"abandoning responsibility for our children"**.

> **"Nothing measures the quality of a society better then how it treats its children. Nothing predicts the future of a society better then how it nurtures and educates its children."**

And on how psychiatry moved in on children he states:

"In blaming the child-victim, psychiatry takes the pressure of the parents, the family, the schools, and society. By diagnosing, drugging and hospitalizing children, psychiatry enforces the worst attitudes towards children in our culture today and exonerates those adult institutions that need reform. Psychiatry has been joined by factions within behavioural educational psychology in exonerating the schools and blaming the children. The question asked by John Holt, "Why can't Jonny read?" Has been answered. Because he has a learning disability."

How are we treating our children at the moment? What kind of future are we nurturing? Why do we look at the children and judge how they are behaving without asking why?

The education system worldwide now and especially in the west has been infiltrated by trained "experts" who seem to have a similar view of how children should behave and if they don't fit into the mould they will need to be guided.

From Aldous Huxley's *Brave New World,* chapter 3:

From a neighbouring shrubbery emerged a nurse, leading by the hand a small boy, who howled as he went. An anxious-looking little girl trotted at her heels.

"What's the matter?" asked the Director.

The nurse shrugged her shoulders. "Nothing much," she answered. "It's just that this little boy seems rather reluctant to join in the ordinary erotic play. I'd noticed it once or twice before. And now again today. He started yelling just now..."

"Honestly," put in the anxious-looking little girl, "I didn't mean to hurt him or anything. Honestly."

"Of course you didn't, dear," said the nurse reassuringly. "And so," she went on, turning back to the Director, "I'm taking him in to see the Assistant Superintendent of Psychology. Just to see if anything's at all abnormal."

Other Rockefeller Foundation donations and funding went to:

American Red Cross

International Health Commission

World's first school of Hygiene and Public Health, at Johns Hopkins University

China Medical Board

Department of Industrial Relations

Social Science Research Council

Eugenics Record Office, with the Carnegie Foundation

Supporters of Henry Kissinger

Council on Foreign Relations

Royal Institute of International Affairs in London

Carnegie Endowment for International Peace

Brookings Institution

World Bank

Harvard, Yale, Princeton and Columbia Universities

University of the Philippines, Los Baños

McGill University

Montreal Neurological Institute

University of Lyon, France

Library of Congress

Bodleian Library at Oxford University

Population Council of New York

Social Science Research Council

National Institute of Public Health of Japan

Group of Thirty

National Bureau of Economic Research

London School of Economics

Trinidad Regional Virus Laboratory

Agriculture and The Green Revolution

The Bellagio Center

Rockefeller Foundation Communication for Social Change Network which supports grassroots/community-based and international non-governmental organisations, (sounds very much to me like the "common purpose" charity in the UK)

The 100 Resilient Cities initiative

Cultural Innovation Fund

And of course the United Nations.

An estimated $14 billion over the years gets a lot of fingers in many pies and with others like the Carnegie Foundation and the new king of giving, Bill Gates, it seems a lot of the things that run societies are actually being funded by very few individuals trying to put life into their own personal "visions".

A quote from the Rockefeller Foundation Bellagio Center:

> **"Since 1959 The Rockefeller Foundation Bellagio Center has hosted thousands of artists, policymakers, scholars, authors, practitioners, and scientists from all over the world enabling them time and space to work, to learn from each other, and to turn ideas into actions that change the world."**

A look into many of the Rockefeller-funded organisations will show how much influence this one family has on the development of the world society.

Legacy of Modern Medicine

Barbara Starfield MD, MDH, 26 JULY 2000, published in *American Medical Association:*

12 000 deaths/year from unnecessary surgery

7000 deaths/year from medication errors in hospitals

20 000 deaths/year from other errors in hospitals

80 000 deaths/year from nosocomial infections in hospitals

106 000 deaths/year from none error, adverse effects of medications

These total to 225,000 deaths per year from iatrogenic causes. This conservative study, shows modern allopathic doctors as the third biggest killer behind heart disease and cancer in the US and as we will see, who knows how much of those are caused by modern allopathic thinking and treatments?

That is the legacy of this "scientific" method used by "experts". Where is the outrage against modern medicine? Where is the precautionary measure towards modern medicine? Where is the propaganda warning of this killer? How would the world be today using methods of a peasant farmer from Austria? What is the true legacy of modern medical thinking and its practices on our bodies and on our minds? Not really a good reason to be going outside and clapping and hitting pots and pans, now, is it!

Bill & Melinda Gates Foundation

Launched in 2000 and is reported to be the largest private foundation in the world, holding $46.8 billion in assets globally, and whose main goals are to enhance healthcare and reduce extreme poverty, and, in the US, to expand educational opportunities and access to information technology.

So, again, similar to the Rockefeller Foundation and Carnegie Foundation, this is a very rich family whose goals are to help needy people, especially in healthcare. By expanding educational opportunities it seems clear to me they want again to tell people what to think and therefore how to behave and using technology. Search patent "060606" to see what "visions" they may have.

> "This is a large part of the reason that Melinda and I got into philanthropy. One of our first big investments was to an organization called Gavi, the Vaccine Alliance. Since 2000, Gavi and partners have immunized more than 760 million children, saving over 13 million lives. And now, Gavi has a new effort underway to purchase COVID-19 vaccines for lower-income countries as soon as they are available."

So from the off his main project was to vaccinate the whole world, claiming to have saved 13 million lives. How that claim can be proven nobody knows but he said it so I guess it must be true.

"Our resources alone are not enough, so we work to change public policies, attitudes, and behaviors to improve lives."

Again, we see some wanting to change public behaviour, which means changing beliefs.

"We partner with governments and the public and private sectors, and foster greater public awareness of urgent global issues."

So they work with all areas of society to tell us what we need to be afraid of, therefore what actions we need to take to avoid these disasters. Remember, we have seen interviews of Bill Gates on TV telling us all we need to know about the pandemic and how and when we will be out of lockdown. Yes, this private business man holding the world in a lockdown (prison term) until his vaccine comes along to free us all. Bill speaks and all the world's politicians listen, what a guy.

In 2018/19 the WHO top four donors were the USA – $851.6 million, UK – $463.4 million, Bill and Melinda Gates Foundation – $455.3 million and GAVI – $388.7 million.

With Gates behind his Foundation and GAVI, this is basically one man funding and therefore controlling the WHO, and remember the WHO was founded on allopathic thinking and Germ Theory, which was funded into existence by the Carnegie and Rockefeller Foundations through the Flexner Report. It must be clear now that "EVENT 201", which, remember, was funded by the Gates Foundation, the World Economic Forum and the WHO, who had for years been priming us with the inevitable viral outbreak threatening mankind, could easily have the wealth and power to utilise the elite-controlled mainstream media. It is estimated just five companies own over 90% of the world's media, and as the 2008 financial crash has already shown us very clearly, world governments represent big banks and corporations and not people. Bailing out banks and not people clearly shows what their priorities are.

Tony Blair, who, evidence shows, lied about "weapons of mass destruction", was never put on trial and was even rewarded by the rich organisations for his actions that resulted in hundreds of thousands of innocent people being murdered by western military action in Iraq, destroying a country for "regime change", which resulted in western companies going in to take control of the resources and even getting contracts to rebuild the country that had just been destroyed. This war criminal is still doing the rounds and still has a political voice.

So it is clear that a mass media campaign and controlling the government narrative would be easy work and also using those same outlets for promoting the philanthropy of Gates, to paint him as some kind as saviour. If you do some simple research you will see he is a very astute business man and doesn't invest (donate) in things if he is not going to get some kind of return.

According to Wikipedia these are the top organisations that received recorded funding in millions of $ between 2009 and 2015 by the Gates Foundation:

GAVI Alliance	3,152.8
World Health Organization	1,535.1
The Global Fund to Fight AIDS, Tuberculosis and Malaria	777.6
PATH	635.2
United States Fund for UNICEF	461.1
The Rotary Foundation of Rotary International	400.1
International Bank for Reconstruction and Development	340.0
Global Alliance for TB Drug Development	338.4
Medicines for Malaria Venture	334.1
PATH Vaccine Solutions	333.4
UNICEF Headquarters	277.6
Johns Hopkins University	265.4
Aeras	227.6
Clinton Health Access Initiative Inc	199.5
International Development Association	174.7

CARE	166.2
World Health Organization Nigeria Country Office	166.1
Agence Française de Développement	165.0
Centro Internacional de Mejoramiento de Maíz y Trigo	153.1
Cornell University	146.7
Alliance for a Green Revolution in Africa	146.4
United Nations Foundation	143.0
University of Washington Foundation	138.2
Foundation for the National Institutes of Health	136.2
Emory University	123.2
University of California San Francisco	123.1
Population Services International	122.5
University of Oxford	117.8
International Food Policy Research Institute	110.7
International Institute of Tropical Agriculture	104.8

From Microsoft they also have investments in companies like FedEx, United Parcel Service, Walmart, Televisa and many more and when looking at these "philanthropists" it is important to ask, are they donating or are they investing?

Other noted funding is to Imperial College London, to the department "Imperial Network for Vaccine Research". Also in May 2009, Bill and Melinda Gates visited Imperial College London after which the Foundation "awarded grants to several Imperial research programmes, including major projects tackling neglected tropical diseases and HIV". Yes, the same institution that gave us Neil Ferguson, who has also benefited from their funding, has over the years been given tens of millions of pounds by the Gates Foundation and GAVI. The British Government themselves are the largest funder of GAVI and this year during the pandemic GAVI were promised £330 million per year over the next five years by Boris Johnson. On the 5th June 2020 at the Global Vaccine Summit 2020, hosted by UK Prime Minister Boris Johnson, world leaders have pledged US$ 8.8 billion for GAVI, the Vaccine Alliance, far exceeding the target of US$ 7.4 billion.

So let's get things clear, a private business man is working with world governments and is funding mass vaccination programmes around the world which will clearly lead to massive profits for vaccine makers, and as you will see later, especially in line with any SARS-coV-2 vaccine, no liability if things go wrong. Now this may seem to you a good man who has done well financially and wants to give back to the world. Why not indeed? But as we have seen, the agenda to vaccinate the world for the health benefits of mankind has not got science behind it and in fact has a legacy of death and suffering and little if any evidence of improving health. And also who does Mr Johnson think he is giving this man our money without even asking us? It seems he doesn't think he needs our permission for anything.

The Gates Foundation also donates massive amounts of money to Planned Parenthood over the globe, promoting contraception, abortion and emergency contraception as well as other areas of sexual health. In fact Bill Gates Senior, another rich philanthropist, has spent time on the board of Planned Parenthood. Its history goes back to Brooklyn, New York, when in 1916 Margaret Sanger, who had close connections to the American Eugenics Society, opened the first birth control clinic in the US. Later, in 1921 she founded the American Birth Control League which evolved into Planned Parenthood in 1942.

Planned Parenthood's push to reform abortion law is normally pushed as a positive move; for example if it is clear there is a seriously deformed child who simply will not survive and is putting the life of the mother at risk, or maybe when a woman is raped and early intervention, especially before about ten weeks before the human form is created, could save her from massive emotional and psychological pain. These examples are where maybe you could see abortion being used to the benefit of individual women but as always, this is the starting point and the finishing point is very far from the starting line.

When looking at the history of Planned Parenthood and Eugenics and the connections to today's "Reproductive Health" programmes sponsored by Planned Parenthood and the Gates Foundation, there is a feeling that all is not as it seems. After the fall of the Nazis, Eugenics certainly had a bad name; it had an elitist ideology and a belief in an elite race to rule humanity, and that humanity should be culled of the weak and undesirable. Basically through breeding, their vision of how humanity should be structured could be made manifest. Putting themselves above God and Nature is an underestimation to say the least. There is clearly no compassion or what we call humanity in this ideology and it gives the impression they see themselves as farmers of human beings to be used as slaves. Just as cattle farmers want to breed the best stock for their own gains, these people see us as cattle to be bred or culled to fit their own needs and visions.

What people like Bruce Lipton showed, though, was that genes are the way cells hold onto the information of the history and present of that person but they do not control life. Life works through the genes but is not controlled by genes; that control comes down to the perception, and as he showed, belief of the individual. So instead of wanting to improve the human race they are actually deliberately holding us back through controlled education and control of perception through instilling beliefs from a young age. The great thing about this truth, though, is we don't need technology or elite help to positively evolve ourselves, we just need to become aware of how life works and focus on opening our own minds and hearts. Yes, there are clearly massive problems within different cultures who maintain unhealthy beliefs but we have to ask ourselves how many of those beliefs were put in place by a level of people above us all, and whose desire is to control us all.

Eugenics never went away, it was just rebranded and its true agenda is one of population control, control in numbers and control in perfecting the perfect slave, and when Mr Gates gets us all chipped and connects us to **AI** he then has the opportunity to create and control humanity as he desires, the perfection of the slave race through Transhumanism.

It is worth noting that they talk about birth control as if nature doesn't provide a way, well it does and it's been known for centuries or more by primitive people, it is commonly known as the Billings Method. It's safe, effective and teaches young girls, and men, discipline, control, respect and how nature works. By showing a young woman how her body works and the difference between different vaginal discharges she can learn when it is possible to conceive or not. There is a certain discharge a sperm needs to survive in the womb; without this, pregnancy cannot occur as the environment is too hostile for the sperm. Mass education in this fact could change the world for young women and men all over the world without using any body-changing toxic drugs and at the same time teaching us how amazing nature is. This knowledge though gives humanity independence and freedom to control our own lives and that doesn't go down well if you have a master plan to control the world.

Looking at the power of the Rockefeller Foundation and Gates, GAVI and

Microsoft, we can now put these together with the ID 2020 alliance.[14]

> **"Alliance partners share the belief that identity is a human right and that individuals must have "ownership" over their own identity."**

This obviously goes on the presumption that just being a human being is not identity enough.

> **"The ability to prove one's identity is a fundamental and universal human right."**

Think what you will but proving my identity sounds like something right out of a police state.

> **"Over 1 billion people worldwide are unable to prove their identity through any recognized means. As such, they are without the protection of law, and are unable to access basic services, participate as a citizen or voter, or transact in the modern economy."**

So without identity they say we have no **"protection of law"**. Do they mean natural law or maritime law? And since when did we need an identity to access water, grow crops or create energy? Why would anyone want to be a **"citizen"** if in doing so they lose their natural sovereignty and rights? As for voting, why vote for who is going to control you?

"Transact in the modern world"

It seems clear that with the loss of cash and the push to cashless and other ways of trading being increasingly difficult, even bartering, to exist without accepting the global control system that ID 2020 will be a challenge.

From the book *IBM and the Holocaust: The Strategic Alliance between*

---

[14] https://id2020.org/alliance

Nazi Germany and America's Most Powerful Corporation: **"detailing IBM's conscious co-planning and co-organizing of the Holocaust for the Nazis, all micromanaged by its president Thomas J Watson from New York and Paris."**

So we have another American company, IBM, with very close connections to the Nazis and their Eugenics programme, the same IBM that in 1980 Microsoft formed a partnership with to bundle Microsoft operating systems with IBM computers. Now remember, it is Bill Gates who seems to be at the moment the main man in telling nations and medical authorities what the strategic plan is to cope with the alleged pandemic, the same global strategic plan that clearly is resulting in mass early death of the weak and elderly, and as in the case at least in the UK, putting do not resuscitate – DNR – orders on many old, weak and physically and mentally disabled people.

Now if that isn't a cull of the undesirable and a reinvention of the Nazi Eugenics programme I don't know what is.

Another big player we can't really leave out is George Soros; it would need a book alone for his story but we'll focus on now and his "Open Society Foundations". **"George Soros is the founder and chair of the Open Society Foundations. He has given away more than $32 billion of his personal fortune to fund the Open Society Foundations' work around the world."** With $15.2 billion in the last three decades into:

Democratic Practice

Early Childhood and Education

Economic Equity and Justice

Equality and Antidiscrimination

Health and Rights

Higher Education

Human Rights Movements and Institution

Information and Digital Rights

Journalism

Justice Reform and the Rule of Law

As you can see, another rich man's Foundation having massive influence over worldwide policies and social movements, to help push his own "vision", I'm sure. Where there are activists it's a good bet Soros is behind funding it.

They are also heavily active in the "Emergency Response to COVID-19" with the current President Patrick Gaspard stating:

> **"But beyond this initial response, it's time to think long and hard about the kind of world we want to live in. For many of us, the pandemic has underlined the challenges to our globalized world, and to the old ways of running our economies, posed by the existential threat of climate change. The current catastrophe also presents an opportunity—an opportunity to push for fundamental changes needed to build societies that are stronger and more resilient in addressing the challenges to come. I assure you that the Open Society Foundations will be an active participant in this search for a better world to emerge from the trauma of our present horror."**

Again, we have a big worldwide problem needing to be solved and the solutions always include "changes" that come from these rich philanthropists. We have the "globalized world" created by rich men behind closed doors in meetings like the Bilderberg Group and we have the "running of our economies" controlled by international mega-rich bankers with a rigged debt-based money system.

"The existential threat of climate change" which again is allegedly caused by man and **"carbon emissions"**, yet leaves out the big yellow thing in the sky in their calculations. Manmade climate change is the story being pushed out of the UN which will be solved through the "UN agenda 21" agreement.

Remember the cute polar bears close to extinction? Well as it happens they are actually thriving despite "global warming", another psychological operation on manipulating human emotions to pass an agenda. Whatever their honourable published goals are on the surface, this is very clearly a planned agenda to bring about total control of human, and animal activity through one central government. This is Communism by stealth.

Some time spent researching who the funders of the Russian revolution and Lenin were will also show up this corporate influence.

Marxism – Fascism – same bird, different wings.

So who has created the "**trauma of our present horror**"? Could it be the same people who now want to "transform" society to build a new and improved model for the world and its "citizens" where we will live in accordance with their "vision"?

I think the Rockefeller – Gates – Soros philanthropy needs a thorough, open and transparent investigation live on TV and to the world to show what they are really up to and where they really want to take society, and humanity with it. This "vision" means that just a few men will decide how all of humanity is going to live, allegedly for the benefit of all of us – mainly because they believe we are too stupid to run our own lives. This is Communism and something like is described in Orwell's book *Animal Farm* and we all know how that turned out, and we also know what happened to Old Major the horse when he started slowing down.

This ideology is borne out of Marxism, and Marxism is borne out of Historical Materialism, which in reality just sees human beings as an ant colony that needs to be organised into the most productive and efficient living system to fulfil our material needs. The colony's needs are paramount and an individual's needs or dreams or ideals are not important. Like all colonies they have to be organised and a strict hierarchy put in place and guess who will be at the top of that hierarchy? Well one is thing for sure, it won't be you or me. I'm sure the "pigs" who will be organising this society will be the ones whose "vision" at the moment is putting it all in place, but I'm sure they'll say from their multi-million-pound castles that they are doing it all for us because they are really nice guys. They certainly "do a lot for charity and don't like to talk about it".

MEDICAL DOCTORS

The UK General Medical Council, direct from their website:

Our role

We are an independent organisation that helps to protect patients and improve medical education and practice across the UK.

We decide which doctors are qualified to work here and we oversee UK medical education and training.

We set the standards that doctors need to follow, and make sure that they continue to meet these standards throughout their careers.

We take action to prevent a doctor from putting the safety of patients, or the public's confidence in doctors, at risk.

Every patient should receive a high standard of care. Our role is to help achieve that by working closely with doctors, their employers and patients, to make sure that the trust patients have in their doctors is fully justified.

Duties of a doctor

The duties of a doctor registered with the General Medical Council

Patients must be able to trust doctors with their lives and health. To justify that trust you must show respect for human life and make sure your practice meets the standards expected of you in four domains.

Knowledge, skills and performance

- Make the care of your patient your first concern.
- Provide a good standard of practice and care.
  - Keep your professional knowledge and skills up to date.
  - Recognise and work within the limits of your competence.

Safety and quality

- Take prompt action if you think that patient safety, dignity or comfort is being compromised.
- Protect and promote the health of patients and the public.

Communication, partnership and teamwork

- Treat patients as individuals and respect their dignity.
  - Treat patients politely and considerately.
  - Respect patients' right to confidentiality.
- Work in partnership with patients.
  - Listen to, and respond to, their concerns and preferences.
  - Give patients the information they want or need in a way they can understand.
  - Respect patients' right to reach decisions with you about their treatment and care.
  - Support patients in caring for themselves to improve and maintain their health.
- Work with colleagues in the ways that best serve patients' interests.

Maintaining trust

- Be honest and open and act with integrity.
- Never discriminate unfairly against patients or colleagues.
- Never abuse your patients' trust in you or the public's trust in the profession.

You are personally accountable for your professional practice and must always be prepared to justify your decisions and actions.

PLEASE REMEMBER ALL THESE DUTIES OF A DOCTOR THE NEXT TIME YOU ARE ASKED FOR YOUR CONSENT TO VACCINATE, BE TESTED OR ARE OFFERED OTHER TREATMENTS AND DRUGS, OR IF YOU WANT TO ASK ABOUT ALTERNATIVE NATURAL THERAPIES.

Extracts from the Hippocratic oath:

"I will use those dietary regimens which will benefit my patients according to my greatest ability and judgment, and I will do no harm or injustice to them. Neither will I administer a poison to anybody when asked to do so, nor will I suggest such a course."

"Into whatsoever houses I enter, I will enter to help the sick, and I will abstain from all intentional wrong-doing and harm, especially from abusing the bodies of man or woman, bond or free."

I think maybe a return to the oath would put us in a better position to stay safe and healthy than the Coronavirus Act 2020 which will do harm, injustice and potentially administer poison. And with its powers to enter our homes I think we could do with that protection and boundaries at this moment in time.

THE GLOBAL PANDEMIC – WHAT JUST HAPPENED?

I have tried my best to give you as much information as I can but in a condensed way, to take us through the next chapters on today's events here in the UK and worldwide. I have tried to show that away from the mainstream media and science there is another way to think of disease. I have also tried to show you there are many invested interests of very rich people in maintaining a belief that drugs are needed for human health and to fight disease. I will now try and take you through the events of the pandemic and how it started, and try and show you where humanity may end up if we keep following the men who claim to be "experts" and also claim they can tell us what to believe and how to behave and when.

The main thing is to try and start with a blank piece of paper and just go with the data and the information shown and also do your own research. See if things add up and if they don't, stop, think, question and research some more. Make up your own mind and don't be swayed by the popular opinion, the "experts" and especially me. Find your own truth and come to your own conclusions. The aim of this book is to open up people's minds and not just ingrain my own personal belief so you exchange one lot of nonsense for another.

So the story begins of the greatest threat to mankind. A story that doesn't begin in China, but in New York.

EVENT 201 – YOUTUBE "Event 201 Pandemic Exercise"

"Event 201" is a pandemic table top exercise hosted by The Johns Hopkins Center for Health Security in partnership with the World Economic Forum and the Bill and Melinda Gates Foundation on October 18, 2019, in New York, NY. The exercise illustrated the pandemic preparedness efforts needed to diminish the large-scale economic and societal consequences of a severe pandemic. Drawing from actual events, Event 201 identifies important policy issues and preparedness challenges that could be solved with sufficient political will and attention. These issues were designed in a narrative to engage and educate the participants and the audience."

– Dr Michael Ryan, Executive Director WHO Health Emergencies Programme

This is the beginning of his introduction:

"The issues we will be dealing with over the next hours may be table top exercises today but they address real and critical threats which we at WHO take very seriously. Without a question epidemic risk has become a Global Strategic Concern. I don't think we've ever been in a situation where we have had to respond to so many health emergencies at once. This is the NEW NORMAL. I don't expect the frequency of these epidemics to reduce and in fact vulnerabilities all over the world in developed and developing countries have increased not decreased, driven by many factors mainly through human behaviour, economic development, population densities and many others. The scenario you will be presented with this morning could easily become one shared reality one day. I fully expect that we will be confronted by a fast moving and highly lethal pandemic of a respiratory pathogen."

What was the scenario they were presented with? An outbreak of coronavirus.

Extract from "epilogue chapter 4":

"The outcome of the CAPS (Coronavirus Associated Pulmonary Syndrome) pandemic in Event 201 was catastrophic. 65 million people dead in the first 18 months. The outbreak was small at first and initially seemed controllable but then it started spreading in densely crowded and impoverished neighbourhoods of mega cities. From that point on the spread of the disease was explosive. Within 6 months cases were occurring in nearly every country."

From WHO website:

WHO Statement regarding cluster of pneumonia cases in Wuhan, China

9 January 2020

Statement

China

Chinese authorities have made a preliminary determination of a novel (or new) coronavirus, identified in a hospitalized person with pneumonia in Wuhan. Chinese investigators conducted gene sequencing of the virus, using an isolate from one positive patient sample. Preliminary identification of a novel virus in a short period of time is a notable achievement and demonstrates China's increased capacity to manage new outbreaks.

Initial information about the cases of pneumonia in Wuhan provided by Chinese authorities last week – including the occupation, location and symptom profile of the people affected – pointed to a coronavirus (CoV) as a possible pathogen causing this cluster. Chinese authorities subsequently reported that laboratory tests ruled out SARS-CoV, MERS-CoV, influenza, avian influenza, adenovirus and other common respiratory pathogens.

Coronaviruses are a large family of viruses with some causing less-severe disease, such as the common cold, and others more severe disease such as MERS and SARS. Some transmit easily from person to person, while others do not. According to Chinese authorities, the virus in question can cause severe illness in some patients and does not transmit readily between people.

Globally, novel coronaviruses emerge periodically in different areas, including SARS in 2002 and MERS in 2012. Several known coronaviruses are circulating in animals that have not yet infected humans. As surveillance improves more coronaviruses are likely to be identified.

China has strong public health capacities and resources to respond and manage respiratory disease outbreaks. In addition to treating the patients in care and isolating new cases as they may be identified, public health officials remain focused on continued contact tracing, conducting environmental assessments at the seafood market, and investigations to identify the pathogen causing the outbreak.

In the coming weeks, more comprehensive information is required to understand the current status and epidemiology of the outbreak, and the clinical picture. Further investigations are also required to determine the source, modes of transmission, extent of infection and countermeasures implemented. WHO continues to monitor the situation closely and, together with its partners, is ready to provide technical support to China to investigate and respond to this outbreak.

The preliminary determination of a novel virus will assist authorities in other countries to conduct disease detection and response. Over the past week, people with symptoms of pneumonia and reported travel history to Wuhan have been identified at international airports.

WHO does not recommend any specific measures for travellers. WHO advises against the application of any travel or trade restrictions on China based on the information currently available.

So, initially, we have someone ill in hospital with pneumonia and the isolation of a novel virus and sequences of the genetic code. No other usual suspects virus-wise seemed to be present indicating this to be the cause. This new virus was said to cause severe illness in some but did not easily spread between people.

It is well documented that main factors in pneumonia are poverty, air pollution, malnutrition, poor sanitation and that the gap between rich and poor countries is great. Surprisingly, China comes out low in the countries with mortality from pneumonia and especially influenza. Some extracts from the 2019 Caixin Global article "Why Aren't People in China Dying of the Flu?"[15] may provide a clue:

> In 2016 and 2017, China reported only 56 and 41 deaths respectively, according to NHC data.
>
> Meanwhile, the U.S. — which counts deaths by flu season, rather than year — saw an <u>estimated 51,000 deaths</u> in the 2016-2017 flu season,

---

[15] https://www.caixinglobal.com/2019-02-21/why-arent-people-in-china-dying-of-the-flu-101382286.html

according to the country's Centers for Disease Control and Prevention (CDC).

One possible reason for China's unusually low flu death numbers is that health officials in the country depend on reports of deaths for their data, rather than the statistical modelling used by authorities elsewhere in the world.

The number of deaths provided by Chinese authorities this week is "likely to be reported deaths in patients with influenza, which will massively underestimate influenza deaths, because most patients in hospitals in China are not tested for influenza," Ben Cowling, a professor at the Hong Kong University School of Public Health, told Caixin. Additionally, not all cases may be reported to the authorities.

"I would predict that more than 100,000 people in China have died from influenza or the complications following influenza virus infection this winter," Cowling said, citing previous studies on flu mortality.

Additionally, doctors in China tend to attribute flu-related deaths to the underlying conditions or complications that make patients more vulnerable to the influenza virus, rath Li Dongzeng, deputy director of the infectious disease center at Beijing You'an Hospital, told Caixin after the 2017 flu season that he believed it was inaccurate to attribute the deaths of patients to the flu if there were other factors at play, like pneumonia or heart disease, which occur commonly in high-risk groups.er than the flu itself.

Medical professionals have argued that not attributing deaths to influenza isn't just a question of statistics and may have a harmful real-world impact.

"The general perception that seasonal influenza does not cause substantial mortality in China may contribute to the underutilization of influenza vaccines in the country," according to a 2012 World Health Organization (WHO) bulletin authored by a team of Chinese and U.S. researchers.

The World Health Organization considers flu vaccines the most effective protection against severe bouts of the flu, and recommends annual vaccination by people at risk, including older and pregnant people, as well as young children.

But a relatively small percentage of the Chinese population gets vaccinated against the flu each year — only 2% in 2018, according to the state-run People's Daily. In contrast, around <u>44% of people in the U.S.</u> were vaccinated against the flu by mid-November 2018, according to the CDC.

So here we can see a theme that is present throughout the book: how can we define an illness? Can we define an illness by the microorganism or viral particle present? This is in fact the biggest question we need to look at. As you can see, defining an illness will bring statistics to life.

Does China really have low influenza rates? If so, why? Does the western world really have high influenza rates and if so, why? With high uptake on influenza vaccines why does the west still have high rates of mortality? With low influenza vaccine rates why does China have low mortality? Why does China take into account underlying conditions more so than the west? Who is right and who is wrong?

Data from an article from the BMJ, PETER DOSHI, DEC 10 2005:

USA 2001 62,034 DEATHS FROM COMBINED PNEUMONIA AND FLU

61,777 PNEUMONIA

257 FLU

ONLY 18 OF WHICH WERE CLINICALLY TESTED AS POSITIVE FOR INFLUENZA VIRUS

USA 1979-2001 AVERAGE OF 1,348 FLU ONLY DEATHS (257-3006)

So, again, we have all the mass hysteria about getting your annual flu jab yet hardly anyone seems to be dying of it, it being the influenza viral particles they say are in circulation, yet seem not to be, or are they but again the classification is wrong, or the test or the doctors' opinion? If in the USA the death rate from influenza is low then why in other papers it is said to be high, and that China is low yet it is really high, but they don't know or test right. Confusion seems to be accepted by the scientific community and they don't seem to be questioning the obvious: what is the flu?

This extract is from an article by James Griffiths, July 11th 2019, for CNN:

China has made major progress on air pollution. Wuhan protests show there's still a long way to go. At 146 globally on the AirVisual list, Wuhan, in northeastern China, is not among China's most polluted cities, but residents aren't taking any chances. Recent weeks have seen major protests there – in themselves a rarity in China – over plans for a new garbage incineration plant.

Holding banners with slogans such as "we don't want to be poisoned, we just need a breath of fresh air," thousands of people took to the city's streets over two weeks in June and July calling for the suspension of plans to build the plant.

"We are fearful that the plant is too close to residence area," one protester in the city of 10 million people told state media. Others expressed concern that emissions could worsen air pollution and harm residents' health.

Local officials were apparently surprised by the scale and size of the protests, which came after several similar waste plants were reportedly found to be giving off dangerous emissions. Photos and videos shared on social media showed large crowds marching in the streets near where the plant was to be built, and police arresting numerous protesters.

The government has since suspended building of the plant, which locals said had halted protests, but a heavy police presence remains in the city where the situation is tense.

So it is clear that the residents in Wuhan were worried about pollution and toxicity in the environment. Wuhan is the largest city in central China with a population of over 11 million. Well known for its steel industry and now 5 car manufacturers, and is an industrial centre in China. The article also shows China along with India having the worst deaths attributable to air pollution in 2017. So does it surprise you that people living in a heavily polluted country and in fact in one of the industrial centres, already protesting about pollution and the environment, in the presence of what history has shown to be a ruthless Communist government (remember "tank man"), may come down with an illness with breathing difficulties as a main symptom?

Why the obsession with finding a new virus as the cause of illness? Why is there zero holistic thinking into the issues of illness and disease coming from the medical authorities, the self-proclaimed "experts"? We all saw the pictures coming out of China, the mayhem, the ruthless control, the madness of people in laboratory protection gear disinfecting whole streets, and people. Is this sheer stupidity, a total lack of awareness or something more sinister? It may be a mixture of all of the above.

Note

On finishing the booklet, China has now totalled 4,634 COVID deaths (6/9/2020). Now you can say that it is so low because of the strict lockdown but that doesn't go well when compared to Peru, as we'll see. With a population of 1,439,323,776 people and massive megacities that is very surprising, it will be even more surprising if they even go above average deaths for the year. Not much of a pandemic so far.

THE SCIENTIFIC METHOD

Let's first just have a look into the scientific method used in China and then the rest of the world which brought them to the conclusion that it was a virus that was passing from person to person, killing all these people.

First it was noted that a number of people were coming down with a severe flu-like issue that manifested in severe breathing difficulties in a wet market. The "experts" took samples, then out of the samples looked for the culprit, assuming it had to be a virus – they do that a lot. How many times have you been to the doctors feeling under the weather and been told "it must be a bug/virus going around"? Hardly a deep investigation and not an ounce of proof needed. They don't really know so it must therefore be a virus.

So they took the samples and found the enemy. They managed to filter out and isolate a virus previously unknown to them, though it has been highly contested by many doctors and scientists that they have not purified a viral particle but just filtered out some genetic material they believe is from an individual particle. So now, without any more tests they have found the enemy; they presume it is new and wasn't there before so in that case it must be the cause.

Science, though, tells us we must look at all information and all factors when doing our best to come to some sort of conclusion. So the obvious information left out is first, what about the physical, energetic and emotional environment of the patients and what else was found in the samples of tissue taken from the patients? Obvious things to look for would be toxins in the environment and if the same toxins are found in the samples, what other influences are in the environment and what other toxins and waste, whether from the outer world or inner cellular waste, is in the samples? This, you would think would be a proper scientific method to at least have a good idea of what is going on and what the influences are on the patient to make them ill or die. This is what we would call holistic thinking, something that has no room in the world of modern medicine.

So, in my opinion, from the start it was not at all a real thorough scientific investigation and the conclusion they came to was not a scientific conclusion. Also, just think about it for a moment, they say they found a new "novel virus" in the patients, but newly found does not mean new as in it has just come into existence. Imagine I go to the Amazon jungle and find, say, a new species of frog, something that does happen. Just finding and identifying that new frog does not mean it has just come into existence; it could have lived there in peace for thousands if not millions of years. Newly discovered does not mean new.

Another observation is that every time a house is on fire you will see a fire engine; they came, though, after the fire started and came with the intention of putting the fire out. I think it would be totally unfair and against British law of "innocent until proven guilty" to blame firemen for starting fires.

Science is just an observation and then asking the questions – why and how did that happen? It doesn't have to take place in a lab and you don't need a white coat and a degree in anything to be scientific. Anyone can be scientific; in fact most of us do make scientific observations every day. We all have the right to observe and think and come to our own conclusions. Don't think you should leave it to the "experts" to tell you what to think and let them tell you their version of events is more accurate than yours because they have letters after their name and use words that most of us don't understand. Look at all observations around an event and bring in all factors and the maybe, just maybe, you may be able to come up with a reasonable idea of why and how.

Medical science and science are not the same thing.

Dr Andrew Kaufman

YouTube – "A Breakdown on Current Testing Procedures"[16]

Here is his take on what was done. What did they do to prove a virus? He says they tested only 7 patients initially.

1. Collect bronchoalveolar (lung) fluids and other samples.

2. Find and separate genetic material from the sample.

---

[16] https://www.youtube.com/watch?v=8kpVGlO5pj8

3. Sequence the genetic material.

4. Rapidly developed a qualitative PCR detection (diagnostic test).

Then he asked these questions:

What about purifying the virus first?

Where did the genetic material come from?

The fact that he says the virus was not purified we know is very relevant as he mentions there is a lot of free genetic material in our bodies at any given time, from bacteria to our own sources like exosomes, so he then goes on to say that without really proving anything they went straight on to devise a test. He explains this here:

COVID-19 RT-OCR Test. Tests for RNA sequence, not the virus.

There is no gold standard

- COVID-19 has never been purified and visualized

- Only visualized from one patient inside a human cell

- RT-PCR never tested against a gold standard

Thus accuracy of test unknown (estimated 80% false positive rate).

Did they isolate a virus or genetic material?

I think Dr Kaufman is right but I'm not a scientist so make up your own mind.[17]

> REUTERS July 3 2020:
>
> **Fact check: Inventor of method used to test for COVID-19 didn't say it can't be used in virus detection**
>
> The context around the quote shows Lauritsen is not saying PCR tests do not work. Instead, he is clarifying that PCR identifies substances qualitatively not quantitatively, detecting the genetic sequences of viruses, but not the viruses themselves: "PCR is intended to identify substances qualitatively, but by its very nature is unsuited for

---

[17] The original scientific paper from Wuhan:
https://www.nejm.org/doi/full/10.1056/nejmoa2001017

estimating numbers. **Although there is a common misimpression that the viral load tests actually count the number of viruses in the blood, these tests cannot detect free, infectious viruses at all; they can only detect proteins that are believed, in some cases wrongly, to be unique to HIV. The tests can detect genetic sequences of viruses, but not viruses themselves.**

So here we see the test does not test for a virus but the genetic sequence believed to be from the virus and it cannot test for viral load, not exactly accurate especially as they didn't purely isolate the virus first.

Dr Kaufman then goes on to show that the alleged COVID-19 virus, SARS-CoV-2, is actually identical to an exosome in every way. As he has shown, these are produced by our own cells when under toxic stress to possibly absorb the toxins, so they are here to help and are not the cause of illness. He also presented photos to show how they even look identical under an electron microscope.

So as we can see no investigation into the environment was included in the conclusion, no other waste or toxic material was looked at in the samples to see what other factors could be involved, and the alleged virus was not passed through Koch's Postulates to show it could cause disease. As the virus was not purely isolated then how do we know what is being tested for? Are the tests actually testing for exosomes, viral particles from our own malfunctioning cells in the form of genetic waste bags, or an alleged invasive virus? Not very clear, is it?

Or as former doctor Parick Quanten puts it:

PCR test does not identify viruses

PCR test has not been standardised and results are therefore not comparable.

The origin of the detected genetic material has not been established.[18]

Think for a moment about the word "isolated". You could isolate a prisoner in a cell; he is isolated, meaning there he is and we can see him. But he may be in the cell with another prisoner or there may be a mouse

---

[18] http://activehealthcare.co.uk/index.php/literature/science/210-pcr-test-what-why-how

in there or flies and spiders. So any information taken out of that cell would include the information of not only your "isolated" prisoner but all else that is in there.

How would you know what information came from where?

I think we need to look at the term "purely isolated" as this would mean it is the prisoner and absolutely nothing else, therefore any information taken out would belong to that prisoner and that prisoner alone. Big difference.

Reliability of antibody and PCR tests

Measles notifications (confirmed cases) England and Wales 1995-2013 by quarter. The table below shows only the cases confirmed by oral fluid IgM antibody tests and/or PCR in each quarter compared to the number of notified cases.[19]

My notes:

Over a four-year period doctors' notifications of measles which ended in a positive test with antibody or PCR method ranged from 1% to 32.7% with an average positive result of 17.68%. Either doctors are mainly wrong in their "guess" or the test is very inaccurate. With false positives and false negatives these tests really don't tell us much. Either way, considering these are the tests that are deciding how much freedom you have or even if you and/or your children can be taken away for further investigation and isolated, it certainly gives rise to many injustices, and also remember, at the moment it is these "positive cases" which are keeping this alleged pandemic alive. On writing this, the UK has been below average deaths for now seven weeks; the show is over, folks, yet we continue with the madness.

---

[19] Source: Notifications of Infectious Diseases confirmed by salivary antibody detection at the Health Protection Agency, Centre for Infections.
(http://www.hpa.org.uk/web/HPAweb&HPAwebStandard/HPAweb_C/1195733811358)

| | | | Tested | | Confirmed | |
Year	Quarter	Uncorrected Notified Cases	Number	%	Number	%
2013*1	4th	535#	620	116.0%	17	2.7%
2013*1	3rd	872	770	88.3%	83	10.8%
2013*1	2nd	3167	2654	83.8%	402	15.1%
2013*1	1st	2222	1369	61.6%	383	28.0%
2012*	4th	1664	944	56.7%	309	32.7%
2012	3rd	1307	873	66.8%	241	27.6%
2012	2nd	1192#	1454	121.9%	419	28.8%
2012	1st	982#	1277	130%	168	13.2%
2011	4th	451#	627	139.0%	138	22.0%
2011	3rd	477#	610	127.8%	154	25.2%
2011	2nd	862#	1208	140.1%	346	28.6%
2011	1st	538#	722	134.2%	151	20.9%
2010	4th	370#	458	123.8%	31	6.8%
2010	3rd	579#	646	111.6%	134	20.7%
2010	2nd	736	641	87.1%	71	11.1%
2010	1st	543	452	83.2%	13	2.9%
2009	4th	519	398	76.7%	4	1.0%
2009	3rd	830	558	62.2%	86	11.1%
2009	2nd	2133	1811	84.9%	482	26.6%
2009	1st	1781	1704	95.7%	304	17.8%

[1] England only data

* Provisional

\# Oral fluid specimens were submitted early from suspected cases and may not have been subsequently notified, thus the proportion tested is artificially high in this quarter.

Another thing to mention is that the sensitivity of the tests can be prepared beforehand. This means you could have an outbreak of many positive tests, "cases", depending on how the tests were calibrated. So if the sensitivity of the tests can be altered then that would leave it wide open to be used for political purposes if people were inclined to do so. Basically "outbreaks" could be created at will.

BBC NEWS 6 SEPT 2020

"Coronavirus: Tests 'could be picking up dead virus'"

The main test used to diagnose coronavirus is so sensitive it could be picking up fragments of dead virus from old infections, scientists say.

Most people are infectious only for about a week, but could test positive weeks afterwards. Researchers say this could be leading to an over-estimate of the current scale of the pandemic. But some experts say it is uncertain how a reliable test can be produced that doesn't risk missing cases.

Prof Carl Heneghan, one of the study's authors, said instead of giving a "yes/no" result based on whether any virus is detected, tests should have a cut-off point so that very small amounts of virus do not trigger a positive result. He believes the detection of traces of old virus could partly explain why the number of cases is rising while hospital admissions remain stable.

Prof Peter Openshaw at Imperial College London said PCR was a highly sensitive "method of detecting residual viral genetic material".

Remember, this is the test they are using to decide if you are at risk of getting ill or making somebody else ill. The results of the test will decide what action follows and if the result is positive then as we will see later it gives Public Health England total power over your life and even your body. Remember, again, it tests for genetic material that we still do not actually know the origin of and yet a whole "track and trace" system has been set up to follow this material. And they are only testing for about 1% of any alleged genome of an alleged virus, a primer.

Dr Stephan Lanka, who is a Virologist, is again challenging the scientific world as to the nature of these alleged viruses. Through "Project

Immanuele" he aims to show the world what scientists are actually doing to prove the existence of these viruses.

> "Virologists have never isolated a complete genetic strand of a virus and displayed it directly, in its entire length. They always use very short pieces of nucleic acids, whose sequence consists of four molecules to determine them and call them sequences. From a multitude of millions of such specific, very short sequences, virologists mentally assemble a fictitious long genome strand with the help of complex computational and statistical methods. This process is called alignment. The result of this complex alignment, the fictitious and very long genetic strand, is presented by virologists as the core of a virus and they claim to have thus proven the existence of a virus."
>
> **Virologists who claim disease-causing viruses are science fraudsters and must be prosecuted.**[20]
>
> – Dr Stephan Lanka

Dr Andrew Kaufman MD and Dr Tom Cowan MD with Sally Farron Morell MA are making the same challenges to the medical science community in the USA. This is part of their statement similar to what other brave doctors have now stated. It will take many more brave doctors to come out and speak this truth to make a difference but the first dominoes are now falling. This truth is what will free us from this invisible attack that is controlling our lives. The whole basis of the lockdown is a PCR test and nobody knows what it's testing for, except some fragments of genetic material all based on a picture of a blob from an electron microscope. It may seem incredible that this is the truth and yet so many "experts" cannot see it at all but hopefully this will be explained later on when we go into the power of beliefs and how they control our perception. Clearly thousands of doctors around the world are not knowingly lying to the public, they just cannot see what is there, hidden in plain sight.

Is this really about tracking a virus or tracking us?

---

[20] https://wissenschafftplus.de/uploads/article/wissenschafftplus-virologists.pdf

Statement On Virus Isolation (SOVI)

Isolation: The action of isolating; the fact or condition of being isolated or standing alone; separation from other things or persons; solitariness.

- Oxford English Dictionary

The controversy over whether the SARS-CoV-2 virus has ever been isolated or purified continues. However, using the above definition, common sense, the laws of logic and the dictates of science, any unbiased person must come to the conclusion that the SARS-CoV-2 virus has never been isolated or purified. As a result, no confirmation of the virus' existence can be found. The logical, common sense, and scientific consequences of this fact are:

the structure and composition of something not shown to exist can't be known, including the presence, structure, and function of any hypothetical spike or other proteins;

the genetic sequence of something that has never been found can't be known; "variants" of something that hasn't been shown to exist can't be known;

it's impossible to demonstrate that SARS-CoV-2 causes a disease called Covid-19.

Sally Farron Morell, MA

Dr Andrew Kaufman, MD

Dr Tom Cowan, MD[21]

---

[21] Full statement found at https://www.andrewkaufmanmd.com

THE FIRST WAVE

Italy

The "virus" was first confirmed to have spread to Italy on 31st January 2020, when two Chinese tourists in Rome tested positive. One week later an Italian man repatriated back to Italy from the city of Wuhan, China, was hospitalised and confirmed as the third case in Italy.

Lombardy

The Lombardy outbreak came to light when a 38-year-old Italian tested positive in Codogno, a commune in the province of Lodi. On 14th February, he felt unwell and went to see a doctor in Castiglione d'Adda. He was prescribed treatments for influenza. On 16th February, as the man's condition worsened, he went to Codogno Hospital, reporting respiratory problems. Initially there was no suspicion of COVID-19, so no additional precautionary measures were taken, and the virus was able to infect other patients and health workers. On 19th February, the wife of the patient revealed he had met an Italian friend who had returned from China on 21st January, who subsequently tested negative. Later, the patient, his pregnant wife and a friend tested positive. On 20th February, three more cases were confirmed after the patients reported symptoms of pneumonia.

Thereafter, extensive screenings and checks were performed on everyone that had possibly been in contact with or near the infected subjects. It was subsequently reported that the origin of these cases had a possible connection to the first European local transmission that occurred in Munich, Germany, on 19th January 2020.

Doctors in Codogno stated that the 38-year-old patient led an active social life in the weeks before his illness and potentially interacted with dozens of people before spreading the virus at their hospital.

An interesting story, but one that cannot be proved.

On 22nd February, the government announced a new decree imposing the quarantine of more than 50,000 people from 11 municipalities in Northern Italy. The quarantine zones are called the Red Zones and the areas in Lombardy and Veneto outside of them are called the Yellow Zones. Penalties for violations range from a €206 fine to three months of imprisonment. The Italian military and law enforcement agencies were instructed to secure and implement the lockdown.

March 9th in the evening, Conte announced in a press conference that all measures previously applied only in the so-called "red zones" had been extended to the whole country, putting approximately 60 million people in lockdown. Conte later proceeded to officially sign the new executive decree.

Confirmed COVID-19 cases in Italy by gender and age

	Classification	Cases Number	Cases (%)	Deaths Number	Deaths (%)	Lethality (%)
All		230,811	(100.0)	31,676	(100.0)	(13.7)
Sex	Male	106,035	(45.9)	18,744	(59.2)	(17.7)
	Female	122,535	(54.1)	12,932	(40.8)	(10.4)
Age	Above 90	18,602	(8.1)	5,415	(17.1)	(29.1)
	80–89	40,532	(17.6)	12,980	(41)	(32)
	70–79	33,141	(14.4)	8,562	(27)	(25.8)
	60–69	30,880	(13.4)	3,259	(10.3)	(10.6)
	50–59	41,435	(18.0)	1,109	(3.5)	(2.7)
	40–49	29,942	(13)	273	(0.9)	(0.9)
	30–39	17,934	(7.8)	62	(0.2)	(0.3)
	20–29	12,933	(5.6)	12	(0.0)	(0.1)
	10–19	3,442	(1.5)	0	(0.0)	(0.0)
	0–9	1,919	(0.8)	4	(0.0)	(0.2)
	n/d	51	(0.0)	0	(0.0)	(0.0)

Source: analysis by *Istituto Superiore di Sanità*[22] on partial set of data, as of 2020/05/26.

Total Coronavirus Deaths in Italy

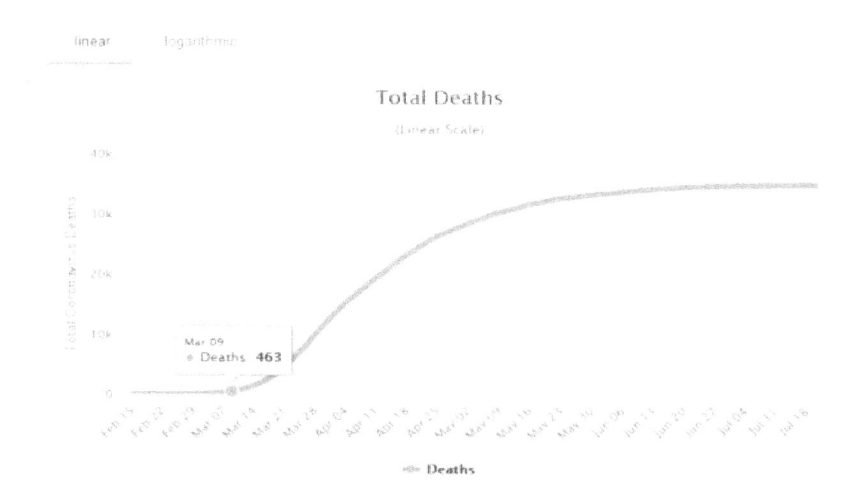

Graph from worldometers

Notice the sharp rise in "coronavirus" deaths occurred AFTER the strict lockdown, a common theme as we shall see as we go on, and that the vast majority were elderly people and children didn't seem to be affected at all.

The centre of the outbreak was Lombardy, a region with a population of about 10 million people, in the industrial centre of Italy and well known for its pollution being some of the worst in Europe. It is also worth noting Italy is well known to have a high percentage of elderly in the population which will become a clear factor in what is happening.

Information from an article in Bloomberg:

---

[22] https://en.wikipedia.org/wiki/Istituto_Superiore_di_Sanita

Italy Says 96% of Virus Fatalities Suffered From Other Illnesses – Tommaso Ebhardt and Marco Bertacche May 26, 2020.

Italy Coronavirus Deaths
Percentage of patients by prior illnesses

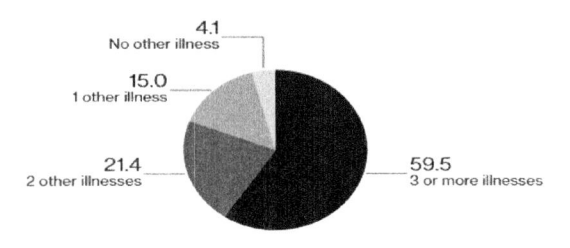

- 4.1 No other illness
- 15.0 1 other illness
- 21.4 2 other illnesses
- 59.5 3 or more illnesses

Source: Italian National Health Institute, May 21 sample of 3,032 deceased

The article which gets data from Italy's ISS health institute also shows just 1.1% of fatalities were from people under 50 years old. That though the average age of a virus case was 62 years old, the average death age was 80 years old. That 30% infected were under 50 years old and 57% of fatalities were 80 years old. 68% had high blood pressure. About 30% diabetes. 28% heart disease.

The Telegraph Online, March 23rd 2020, Professor Walter Ricciardi, scientific adviser to Italy's minister of health said:

> "**the way in which we code deaths in our country is very generous in the sense that all the people who die in hospitals with the coronavirus are deemed to be dying of the coronavirus.**"
>
> "**On re-evaluation by the National Institute of Health, only 12 per cent of death certificates have shown a direct causality from coronavirus, while 88 per cent of patients who have died have at least one pre-morbidity - many had two or three.**"

So, again, why is the medical thinking just to blame a "virus" when clearly there were many factors involved? It seems that children and middle aged people especially with no health issues were at no risk at all and "no other illnesses" should really read "no known illnesses", as many people can have no symptoms of illness but disease can be building up in their body without knowing.

Former doctor Patrick Quanten has said many times before that many people will have cancer maybe six times or so in their lives without it manifesting into a full-blown obvious tumour, so without a thorough investigation it is hard to say if there were no other factors in all deaths.

With the aged population in Italy well known and all the other health issues, it was something that was bound to happen one day, a year, or maybe two or three with a large proportion of elderly deaths. Again, we saw the horrific pictures of hysteria, control, panic and death raging in Italy coming out of the mainstream news, all blamed on this new "virus" out of China which was on a warpath to destroy us all.

Again, where was the calm and rational holistic thinking?

A common theme is the medical profession saying that the rise in deaths started with the lockdowns because they caught the "virus" just at the right time, and if it wasn't for the lockdown timing things would have been worse. Great to have a story you can't prove and even more incredible is this not-alive, non-moving "virus" that can seem to coordinate its attack just at the time of lockdowns.

Spain

Knowing the global policy for dealing with the outbreak of the virus, we only really need to look at the data.

On the 7th March the area of Haro was put into lockdown, then on the 12th of March the Catalan regional government quarantined four municipalities due to a cluster of cases. A national state of emergency was declared on 14th March 2020 which effectively put Spain into lockdown and people were told to go home and on 30th March, it was announced that, beginning the following day, all non-essential workers were ordered to remain at home initially for the next 14 days. The lockdown was strictly enforced by the police and strict social distancing was put in place. March 14th, day of lockdown, there had been 196 "COVID" deaths.

Total Coronavirus Deaths in Spain

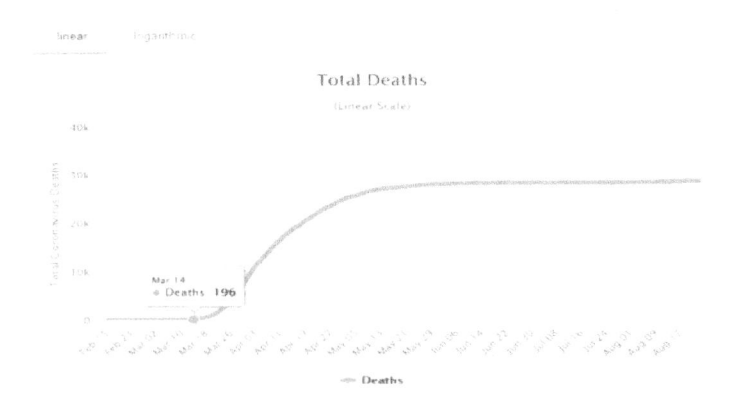

Graph taken from worldometers

Again, notice the pattern of a sharp rise in "coronavirus" deaths after the lockdown. Either the governments of the world were all catching this "virus" just in time and it was coordinating the attack with the lockdown timing, or again, the worldwide lockdown policy was actually killing people, or maybe a bit of both. It could be looked at that yes, the government did intervene at the right time and after about two weeks or so deaths started to drop and that was because of the lockdown and social distancing – that could be argued – but as we will see, with the policies in the UK, it is very clear that the protocols and decision making in stating what was a "COVID" death were global policies.

I have tried to find graphs showing the age range of people dying in Spain but can't seem to find any. From early reports the story seems to follow the same path of mainly elderly with underlying health conditions being the vast majority of people affected. So the scene was set for this insatiable deadly enemy to come over to the UK and like something from World War Two the nation's leaders rose up to the challenge of the coming war.

Terrorism ACT200

Terrorism: interpretation

(1) In this Act "terrorism" means the use or threat of action where—

   a) the action falls within subsection (2),
   b) the use or threat is designed to influence the government [F1or an international governmental organisation] or to intimidate the public or a section of the public, and
   c) the use or threat is made for the purpose of advancing a political, religious [F2, racial] or ideological cause.

(2) Action falls within this subsection if it—

   d) involves serious violence against a person,
   e) involves serious damage to property,
   f) endangers a person's life, other than that of the person committing the action,
   g) creates a serious risk to the health or safety of the public or a section of the public, or
   h) is designed seriously to interfere with or seriously to disrupt an electronic system.

The Enemy Has Landed

GOV.UK, 31/1/2020

Chief Medical Officer, Professor Chris Whitty, statement about cases of novel coronavirus in England.

> **"We can confirm that 2 patients in England, who are members of the same family, have tested positive for coronavirus. The patients are receiving specialist NHS care, and we are using tried and tested infection control procedures to prevent further spread of the virus.**
>
> **The NHS is extremely well-prepared and used to managing infections and we are already working rapidly to identify any contacts the patients had, to prevent further spread. We have been preparing for UK cases of novel coronavirus and we have robust infection control measures in place to respond immediately. We are continuing to work closely with the World Health Organization and the international community as the outbreak in China develops to ensure we are ready for all eventualities."**

> "This is the worst Public health crisis in a generation ... and I must level with you and the British public, more families, many more families, are going to lose loved ones before their time."
>
> – Boris Johnson, 12th March 2020

At that time, 12th March, there had allegedly been 596 cases and ten deaths from the "deadly virus".

We were being repeatedly told that **"at all stages we have been guided by the science, we will do the right thing at the right time"** coming from Mr Johnson, again, and of course Matt Hancock.

Chief Scientific Advisor Sir Patrick Vallance estimated **"that the UK was four weeks behind the trajectory of the crisis in Italy and that the peak might not come for 10-14 weeks running into June."**

Dr Halpern is chief executive of the government-owned Behavioural Insights Team, known as the "nudge unit", and a member of Whitehall's Scientific Advisory Group for Emergencies (Sage) and also co-authored a government document titled "MINDSPACE":

> "If the virus spreads as modelling suggests it will, government advisers believe some hard choices will need to be made about how to protect groups that are more vulnerable to the disease – particularly the 500,000 older people in care homes and those with respiratory conditions."

> "There's going to be a point, assuming the epidemic flows and grows as it will do, where you want to cocoon, to protect those at-risk groups so they don't catch the disease. By the time they come out of their cocooning, herd immunity has been achieved in the rest of the population."

Deputy Chief Medical Officer Jenny Harren:

> "the thing about a new virus is, of course, nobody has antibodies ready-made to it. The virus is having a field day; the desire will be to infect as many people as it can."

So, again, repeating that this virus is "new", we do not have the needed antibodies to protect us – antibodies the WHO know don't correspond to protection, and it has a **"desire** to infect as many people as it can" (again, where that desire comes from no one seems to know).

So the general message is they are using the "best available science" and we need to be afraid, be very afraid. Many of us will die and basically there is nothing we can do except run and hide and hope for the best. The enemy is coming, the invisible beast whose only reason to live is to kill human beings with its insatiable appetite. This message was put out by the government and their array of medical and scientific "experts" and was repeated without any investigation whatsoever by all the mainstream press and media. No health advice was given and we were told we were all possible victims of this monster.

16th March 2020

Imperial College COVID-19 Response Team

Report 9: Impact of non-pharmaceutical interventions (NPIs) to reduce COVID-19 mortality and healthcare demand

Extract taken from introduction:

> The COVID-19 pandemic is now a major global health threat. As of 16th March 2020, there have been 164,837 cases and 6,470 deaths confirmed worldwide. Global spread has been rapid, with 146 countries now having reported at least one case. The last time the world responded to a global emerging disease epidemic of the scale of the current COVID-19 pandemic with no access to vaccines was the 1918-19 H1N1 influenza pandemic.
>
> The report talked about three options.
>
> The first option was no action and no change in public behaviour with an estimated 81% of UK and US population infected with 510 000 deaths in UK and 2.2 million in the US.
>
> Second option was mitigation with an estimated 250 00 deaths in UK and 1.1-1.2 deaths in the US.
>
> The third option was suppression; it is not clear from the report the deaths if suppression was chosen but Azra Ghani, a member of the Imperial team. Was reported to have said that suppression "might bring total deaths down to about 20,000 if they were observed strictly."

Extract taken from summary:

> The global impact of COVID-19 has been profound, and the public health threat it represents is the most serious seen in a respiratory virus since the 1918 H1N1 influenza pandemic. Here we present the results of epidemiological modelling which has informed policymaking in the UK and other countries in recent weeks. In the absence of a COVID-19 vaccine, we assess the potential role of a number of public health measures –so-called non-pharmaceutical interventions (NPIs) – aimed at reducing contact rates in the population and thereby reducing

transmission of the virus. In the results presented here, we apply a previously published microsimulation model to two countries: the UK (Great Britain specifically) and the US. We conclude that the effectiveness of any one intervention in isolation is likely to be limited, requiring multiple interventions to be combined to have a substantial impact on transmission. Two fundamental strategies are possible: (a) mitigation, which focuses on slowing but not necessarily stopping epidemic spread – reducing peak healthcare demand while protecting those most at risk of severe disease from infection, and (b) suppression, which aims to reverse epidemic growth, reducing case numbers to low levels and maintaining that situation indefinitely. Each policy has major challenges. We find that that optimal mitigation policies (combining home isolation of suspect cases, home quarantine of those living in the same household as suspect cases, and social distancing of the elderly and others at most risk of severe disease) might reduce peak healthcare demand by 2/3 and deaths by half. However, the resulting mitigated epidemic would still likely result in hundreds of thousands of deaths and health systems (most notably intensive care units) being overwhelmed many times over. For countries able to achieve it, this leaves suppression as the preferred policy option.

The report ended by saying:

We therefore conclude that epidemic suppression is the only viable strategy at the current time. The social and economic effects of the measures which are needed to achieve this policy goal will be profound. Many countries have adopted such measures already, but even those countries at an earlier stage of their epidemic (such as the UK) will need to do so imminently.

Our analysis informs the evaluation of both the nature of the measures required to suppress COVID-19 and the likely duration that these measures will need to be in place. Results in this paper have informed policymaking in the UK and other countries in the last weeks. However, we emphasise that is not at all certain that suppression will succeed long term; no public health intervention with such disruptive effects on society has been previously attempted for such a long duration of time. How populations and societies will respond remains unclear.

It seems this **"expert"**, Neil Ferguson, is basically a mathematician in a white coat. He doesn't seem to have looked into the historical conditions of the 1918 pandemic and had based all his models on an invisible enemy called a virus transmitting from one person to another. He also seems to have no knowledge of the human experiments conducted by the Public Health Service and the US Navy we showed earlier, where it was shown to be not possible to infect any volunteers with flu passed on by ill patients no matter what they did.

To be clear about these computer-generated models, what you get out depends on what you put in. Crap in, crap out. The "R" rate is from a computer-generated model based on germ/viral theory which we already know is far from being proven correct.

Let's take a look at the history of this man who was chosen as the team "expert" to give us the best information and advice on how to deal with the coming threat.

Professor Neil Ferguson – Imperial College London

[Imperial College epidemiologist Neil] Ferguson worked on the disputed research that sparked the mass culling of eleven million sheep and cattle during the 2001 outbreak of foot-and-mouth disease.[23]

In 2002, Ferguson predicted that between 50,000-100,000 people could die from exposure to BSE (mad cow disease) in beef. In the UK, there were only 178 deaths from BSE.

In 2005, Ferguson predicted that up to 200 million people could be killed from bird flu. Only 282 people died worldwide from the disease between 2003 and 2009.

In 2009, a government estimate based on Ferguson's advice said a "reasonable worst-case scenario" was that the swine flu would lead to 65,000 British deaths. In the end, swine flu killed 457 people in the UK.

(Worldwide the WHO reported only 18,449 deaths from swine flu as of 1/8/2010.[24])

So while all the time the government tells us they are being led by the best available science they take advice from a man with a track record like

---

[23] https://www.youtube.com/watch?v=Yb9iaDoXJF8
[24] https://www.who.int/csr/don/2010_08_06/en/

this. Is this incompetence, stupidity or, again, something more sinister?

When it came to light that 114 files concerning allegations of child abuse had been **"lost or destroyed"**, the contents of which dated from 1979-1999, Home Secretary Teresa May was quoted responding to the Wanless Report's publication, telling MPs:

> **"There might have been a cover-up. I cannot stand here and say the Home Office was not involved in a cover-up in the 1980s and that is why I am determined to get to the truth."**

Was anything done and was there a full investigation and arrests? No, of course not, in fact she was rewarded for her failure by succeeding David Cameron as prime minister in 2016.

Remember Tony Blair giving us the best available science of "weapons of mass destruction", advice that led to the massacre of hundreds of thousands of innocent Iraqis and the total destruction of a nation? A man that to this day is still allowed a political voice.

Remember doctors promoting cigarette smoking and prescribing thalidomide? Again, they were giving the best scientific advice they had.

Remember being told the ice caps are going to melt, the polar bears will all die, the world will be flooded and England will be like the Mediterranean? Well that was thirty years ago and they are still pushing it now; strange they never put that big yellow thing in the sky into their calculations and the polar bears seem to be doing just fine.

The list of bad scientific advice being pushed as fact and impacting badly on human beings would make up a thousand-page book by itself. I hope those few at least start to make you question the latest advice. So with just ten deaths and it seems now, with new evidence, coronavirus has been about for months or even longer before we were told – like I said, the information is changing by the day – we go into lockdown. Another thing to think of is that if it is true, and using their scientific thinking, coronavirus had already been in circulation for months and through the winter, at a time when our resistance is low, what was it doing? Where were the mass deaths?

As you will see, the massive spike in deaths occurred AFTER lockdown; again, as you will see, a common theme. So we go to war, or at least the politicians and their "medical experts" tell us to prepare for war. Our glorious leaders giving us permanent updates of how the enemy is attacking and, I'm not sure about you, but the whole drama with politicians dramatically coming through doors to address the nation was like watching Hitler taking the stand talking to the masses or any other dictator addressing the masses. We, though, were given a vision of him being a new Winston Churchill. Of course, a nation at war and in emergency conditions gives politicians a free-for-all in taking our freedoms away in the name of protecting us and we started to see mass Orwellian doublespeak being used to perfection.

Scary stuff and I'm not talking about the virus.

From GOV.UK website:

Status of COVID-19

As of 19 March 2020, COVID-19 is no longer considered to be a high consequence infectious disease (HCID) in the UK.

The 4 nations public health HCID group made an interim recommendation in January 2020 to classify COVID-19 as an HCID. This was based on consideration of the UK HCID criteria about the virus and the disease with information available during the early stages of the outbreak. Now that more is known about COVID-19, the public health bodies in the UK have reviewed the most up to date information about COVID-19 against the UK HCID criteria. They have determined that several features have now changed; in particular, more information is available about mortality rates (low overall), and there is now greater clinical awareness and a specific and sensitive laboratory test, the availability of which continues to increase.

The Advisory Committee on Dangerous Pathogens (ACDP) is also of the opinion that COVID-19 should no longer be classified as an HCID.

The need to have a national, coordinated response remains, but this is being met by the government's COVID-19 response.

Cases of COVID-19 are no longer managed by HCID treatment centres only. All healthcare workers managing possible and confirmed cases should follow the updated national infection and prevention (IPC) guidance for COVID-19, which supersedes all previous IPC guidance for COVID-19. This guidance includes instructions about different personal protective equipment (PPE) ensembles that are appropriate for different clinical scenarios.

On the 23rd March 2020, four days after COVID-19 was declared not to be a high-consequence infectious disease, the UK went into lockdown, not quarantine, but the prison term of lockdown was used.

> **"From this evening I must give the British people a very simple instruction – you must stay at home."**
>
> – Boris Johnson, after allegedly 6,030 cases and 359 deaths "from COVID".

The Prime Minister announced that the police will now have the power to fine people if they leave their homes for any reason other than the following:

> **Shopping for basic necessities**
>
> **One form of exercise a day – either alone or with members of your household**
>
> **Medical need or to provide care help vulnerable person**
>
> **Travel to work – but only if necessary and you cannot work from home**
>
> **"You should not be meeting friends, you should not be meeting family members who don't live in your home, you should not be shopping except for essentials."**
>
> **"If you don't follow the rules, the police have power to enforce them including with fines."** (Something later declared to be a lie and the fines were unlawful.)
>
> **"Police have also been given extra powers, stopping motorists to check if their journeys are essential."**
>
> **"We will stop all gatherings of more than two people in public and stop all social events."**

For me personally, whilst the whole nation was running around buying toilet rolls and running for cover, I went home and had a cup of tea. Remember the film "Carry On Up The Kyber" when the fort was being bombed and the officers were just in the dining hall having dinner with their wives, all dressed up and going on as though nothing at all was happening, that is the British way. When the shit hits the fan just sit down and have a cup of tea, the British solution to many a problem, or just the best thing to do when there is nothing else you can do.

Here are some examples of madness in the first few weeks. The madness, though, is still continuing to date.

Police screaming at people in the street in London, "Go home. You're killing people."

Police putting a black dye in a lake at an isolated beauty spot in Yorkshire after they filmed and shamed a woman walking her dog in the middle of nowhere with her child.

Police stopping and fining people in their cars just for being on the road or even just walking to work. Something they had no right to do.

Police setting up road blocks to stop people to ask why they are out of their homes.

Police being asked to go into supermarkets to check that what people were buying was all essential stuff.

Police arresting a woman for doing yoga on a bench alone in a London park.

Police telling people on beaches or in parks or even outside their own homes to go in; it's the virus, you know.

The list for the police could go on and on.

There were people at home ranting on social media or shouting out of their windows about someone outside their house or across the street walking his dog and stopping to talk for someone, putting us all in danger.

For years people whingeing on about teenagers in groups in the street taking part in anti-social behaviour, now they are complaining about social behaviour; they can't win either way.

The toilet roll crisis, I've still no idea what that was about.

We were told it was all about "flattening the curve and taking the pressure" off the NHS.

Then all the mad, insane guidelines like, you can visit your mum and dad but one at a time in separate rooms and ten minutes apart, something referred to on one TV programme as "bonkers". Oh, and please "don't sing or shout". All the things you can do and the things you can't, even in your own home, all the contradictions, all the nonsense which we were told was being "guided by the best science". Guidelines changing almost every day, no one really knowing what was going on; different rules in England, Wales, Scotland and Northern Ireland. A total shambles, but I feel it was organised chaos. Chaos creates confusion, confusion means no one can see what is really happening, this way people can be easily controlled. Out of the chaos must come the order and the order was to be the "new normal".

Coronavirus Act 2020

SCHEDULE 21 PART 2 Powers relating to potentially infectious persons in England

Powers to direct or remove persons to a place suitable for screening and assessment

6

(1) This paragraph applies if, during a transmission control period, a public health officer has reasonable grounds to suspect that a person in England is potentially infectious.

(2) The public health officer may, subject to sub-paragraph (3) —

(a) direct the person to go immediately to a place specified in the direction which is suitable for screening and assessment,

(b) remove the person to a place suitable for screening and assessment, or

(c) request a constable to remove the person to a place suitable for screening and assessment (and the constable may then do so).

(3) A public health officer may exercise the powers conferred by this paragraph in relation to a person only if the officer considers that it is necessary and proportionate to do so —

(a) in the interests of the person,

(b) for the protection of other people, or

(c) for the maintenance of public health

(4) Where a public health officer exercises the powers conferred by this paragraph, the officer must inform that person —

(a) of the reason for directing or removing them, and

(b) that it is an offence —

(i) in a case where a person is directed, to fail without reasonable excuse to comply with the direction, or

(ii) in a case where a person is removed (by the officer or by a constable), to abscond.

7

(1) This paragraph applies if, during a transmission control period—

(a) a constable, or

(b) an immigration officer in the course of exercising any of their functions, has reasonable grounds to suspect that a person in England is potentially infectious.

(2) The immigration officer or constable may, subject to sub-paragraph (3) —

(a) direct the person to go immediately to a place specified in the direction which is suitable for screening and assessment, or

(b) remove the person to a place suitable for screening and assessment.

(3) An immigration officer or constable may exercise the powers conferred by this paragraph in relation to a person only if the officer or constable considers that it is necessary and proportionate to do so —

(a) in the interests of the person,

(b) for the protection of other people, or

(c) for the maintenance of public health.

(4) Where an immigration officer or constable exercises the power to direct or remove a person under this paragraph, the officer or constable must inform that person —

(a) of the reason for directing or removing them, and

(b) that it is an offence —

(i) in a case where a person is directed, to fail without reasonable excuse to comply with the direction, or

(ii) in a case where a person is removed, to abscond.

(5) An immigration officer or constable must, before exercising the powers conferred by this paragraph, consult a public health officer to the extent that it is practicable to do so.

Part 10 interested me – **"impose other requirements"** – so vague it is a permission slip to do anything.

10

(6) A public health officer may —

(a) require the person referred to in paragraph 8 to be screened and assessed, and

(b) impose other requirements on the person in connection with their screening and assessment.

Remember, it is an unreliable RCR test that will decide how much freedom you have and how much power PHE have over you and your body.

It is an absolute must that everyone should be reading this "act"; it is pure medical fascism. Where is the "law of consent" here? Basically all rights over your own body are gone and you and your children can be whisked off anywhere they choose. With all the new rules and guidelines to be enforced, how could it possibly done by the police force alone? Easy, get the people to police themselves. Schools were teaching children before the lockdown to tell everyone at home to stop touching their faces, even to shout, "Face!" at their parents when they did. The "educated" children, Hitler Youth, would enforce policy on the parents. The rest would be done by being a "good citizen" and basically telling on your neighbour. Add to that, people in fear shouting at nonconformers in the street. So the sheep would sheep themselves.

As psychologist Professor Jordan Peterson stated, **"you probably would have been a Nazi too"**, when talking about how Nazi Germany came about and why it was all backed by the majority of the public and "men in uniform" just "doing their job". We have the script of George Orwell's *1984* in full flow with plenty of Aldous Huxley's *Brave New World* social engineering thrown in for good measure.

Then surprise, surprise, Boris Johnson "gets it", this deadly disease whose main symptom was a persistent dry cough. He addressed the nation, telling us of his trial with the illness without even coughing once. "Things that make you go hmmmm." After a touch-and-go illness, "nudged" away from public view of course, so we'll just have to take their word for it, our glorious leader came back with more energy for the war than ever and even more energy to tell us what we can and cannot do. It may seem to many that comparing the government propaganda to warlike is over the top but given that now we know the military are being used to actually monitor the population they are sworn to protect, we need to ask, who is the enemy here?

Enter the "77th brigade"

> **"We are a combined Regular and Army Reserve unit. Our aim is to challenge the difficulties of modern warfare using non-lethal engagement and legitimate non-military levers as a means to adapt behaviours of the opposing forces and adversaries."**

So the British Government is joining forces with the British Army to **"adapt behaviours of the opposing forces and adversaries"**. The obvious question here is, who are the **"opposing forces and adversaries"** and what **"behaviour"** needs adapting? Well, considering behaviour is controlled by beliefs – we will come to that later – the question should be, what beliefs are deemed dangerous by the British Government surrounding the "corona pandemic"?

> **"Some of the ways we help"** are **"Collecting, creating and disseminating digital and wider media content in support of designated tasks."**

So it seems clear they are an intelligence unit scanning social media and the like with **"designated tasks"** in mind. So, again, what information are they looking for that would highlight people as possible **"adversaries"**? When targeted, where does this information go? And what is the next step against these **"adversaries"**?

Well, it's clear they are working with government on the information surrounding the "corona pandemic", therefore it would then be clear they are looking for information and people who do not believe the government narrative. I would suggest, then, these are the **"adversaries"** they are looking for.

Also part of what they do under **"Human Security"** is:

> **"Human Security puts the emphasis on security of the people and their social and economic environment rather than focusing on security of the state."**

Doesn't it seem strange to you that a unit in the British Army that is claiming to protect the people and their social and economic security, is actually being used by British politicians who are taking all the freedoms away from the British people; not only destroying but reconstructing all the social interactions and putting into place rules that will no doubt destroy the economy and bankrupt the nation?

Under **"news and events"** they show us more of their activities:

> **"Dispelling rumours. Don't believe everything you read elsewhere, if you want to check what the Army is doing for COVID-19 check here and our social media channels on Twitter, Facebook, LinkedIn and Instagram."**

So they are actively engaging in social media to push the government line and to see who is out there with alternative opinions. If these alternative opinions are so wrong and dangerous then why not have a full public debate and let us see all this "fake news" for what it is?

Just a look at what is happening in Victoria, Australia, shows you how people's Facebook pages are being monitored and people are being arrested or harassed because of their posts questioning the official narrative. If it is so wrong, surely we could all see it for ourselves. This all comes down to control of information and therefore control of truth which leads to control of behaviour.

> **"The Army's priority remains to protect the UK public in these unprecedented times."**

So by protecting us they mean they are making sure we think the "right way". I don't think the enemy has landed; I think it was here all along.

WELCOME TO NAZI BRITAIN AND YOU AIN'T SEEN NOTHING YET.

DEATH BY LOCKDOWN?

Thanks to Ann Leyshon for her research and writing on this most important chapter.

As explained in the previous chapter, there was a sudden rise in excess deaths for all the countries studied only after lockdown was enforced. Additionally, when you look at how the UK compares with the rest of the world, the results are indeed shocking. As the data shows, the UK has the second highest deaths per million in the world. You are around 150 times more likely to die of this virus in the UK than you are in a densely populated country such as India.

The British Medical Journal has also written a paper requesting the urgent address of the fact that only a third of the thousands of excess deaths seen in the community in England and Wales can be explained by COVID-19. Another study has found that the majority of those hospitalised were those who were completely self-isolating as instructed and not going out at all.

Even 'The Guardian' newspaper reported that there were almost 10,000 unexplained extra deaths among people with dementia in England and Wales in April according to official figures that have prompted alarm and raised questions about the severe impact of social isolation on people with the condition.

So what is going on?

If one believes in the virus and the validity of the PCR tests used to identify it, then the virus has been around for at least a year. So what has caused the sudden spike in deaths only after lockdown and such huge discrepancies in excess deaths between countries? This cannot possibly be because of the same alleged virus. This is clearly about lockdown and even more so, the lockdown policies implemented. To properly appreciate the complexities involved, each area will need to be looked at individually.

Care home deaths

By far the biggest impact in Europe of this pandemic was within the care home system. The countries with the highest death rates ALL had a policy of isolating the elderly in these facilities as opposed to ongoing and normal care within communities and families. Around 50% of the deaths occurred within this area.

It is widely acknowledged that the vast majority of those who have died with COVID-19 had at least one serious comorbidity and were over 65 years old with more than 83% over 70. The deaths have occurred almost exclusively among those who were approaching, or already receiving, end-of-life care. It would appear that these deaths within care home facilities were effectively hastened. How could this have happened? What was implemented that could have possibly achieved this result?

The following policies were implemented at the beginning of lockdown in order to "protect the NHS":

1. NHS England decided not to allow specified groups of vulnerable patients to be admitted to hospital. This meant not treating those over the age of 70, who displayed normal vital signs, and any who had supposedly elected not to be resuscitated, regardless of their health condition.

2. Vulnerable and older people both in care homes and within the community were pressured to sign "do not attempt resuscitation" (DNAR) notices. Additionally were numerous reports of these being completed en masse without the older person's consent in care settings, automatically excluding vulnerable people from hospital treatment.

3. Further, the guidance advised that vulnerable people should not be taken to Accident and Emergency departments unless approved by a clinical adviser, thereby increasing the delay in treatment during the vital golden hour. This caused considerable concern amongst health professionals.

While these policies were implemented, all care home visits from family and loved ones were suspended. Residents were isolated and confined to their rooms, routine care and therapies were withdrawn, as was the ability to go outside and exercise. An often-unfamiliar skeleton staff remained who were often barely able to attend to basic needs. This kind of treatment and confinement would highly likely lead to the development of serious life-threatening illnesses and terrible health and mental outcomes. Reduced mobility could cause an elderly person to become constipated and this may push up on the diaphragm and cause atelectasis or cause them to vomit and aspirate leading to pneumonia. Confinement may have caused them to develop urinary retention and UTI, secondary to constipation, and become bedbound, causing more time in a prone position and development of basal collapse of the lungs and again, atelectasis and pneumonia. Just the fact that they had reduced mobility may even mean they spent more time in bed or just sitting, which again, is enough to cause chest infection/pneumonia.

The Mail Online on the 12th July 2020 headlined:

"Did care homes use powerful sedatives to speed Covid deaths?"

They show that through the month of April, out-of-hospital prescription for the drug midazolam, a powerful sedative that can be used to relieve anxiety, pain and stress and if enough is used can provide total sedation to dying patients, went from the average of 15,000 to 38,582, more than double.

They quote retired neurologist Professor Patrick Pullicino as stating:

> **"Midazolam depresses respiration and it hastens death. It changes end-of-life care into euthanasia."** He also said, **"Midazolam depresses respiration and it hastens death. It changes end-of-life care into euthanasia."**

So the question is, what was happening in the care homes that was creating such anxiety, stress and pain? And was midazolam being used in the manner of the infamous "Liverpool Care Pathway", prematurely ending patients' lives?

A small French study labelled what they found as **"confinement disease"**. The April paper concluded that more than 24 deaths at a long-term care facility, that staff believed were due to the virus were actually from hypovolemic shock, a life-threatening condition caused by a rapid loss of blood or fluids. The victims had been confined to their rooms for days with no assistance eating or drinking due to low staff numbers and a lack of personal protective equipment.

More than a month after Shoshana Padro's Toronto nursing home closed to visitors, her daughter Lenore got news that she was barely eating or drinking and was on the verge of death. Lenore Padro had been worried about how her mother would manage without extra help at mealtimes. The 79-year-old, who had dementia and needed to be spoon-fed, always ate more when her daughter or private caregiver visited and had time to coax her to take another bite. The elder Ms. Padro, who twice tested negative for the coronavirus, died on April 28th. Her health had previously been stable, and her daughter believes she died of dehydration or starvation.

Heather Keller, who researches nutrition and ageing at the University of Waterloo, said long-term care residents who eat in their rooms don't consume as much, especially those with cognitive impairments, who lose out on the important social cues they would otherwise get in the dining room. "That's a big part of this, is the lack of that social connectedness at meal times that stimulates food intake for older adults," Prof. Keller said.

Ralf Leswal is haunted by worries that his wife, Karen, who had Huntington's disease, wasn't properly cared for in her final weeks. He used to spend hours every day caring for her at Orchard Villa, her nursing home in Pickering, Ont., including slowly feeding her so that she wouldn't aspirate her food. Ms. Leswal contracted COVID-19 and died on April 30th. **"I wonder, did my wife actually die of COVID or did she die of neglect?"** he said.

"People, we're hearing, are really not eating. Not everyone, but there's a real concern," said Laura Tamblyn Watts, chief executive officer of CanAge, a national seniors advocacy organisation. **"It's incredibly dire."**[25]

Other staff at care homes reported that residents confined to their rooms and forbidden to have visits from loved ones were giving up on life and "fading away". **"The virus won't be the killer of these people, it's the distress and fear of not seeing family that is doing it,"** said one carer who asked to remain anonymous but who reported her concerns to the Care

---

[25] https://www.theglobeandmail.com/canada/article-what-happened-when-families-were-blocked-from-long-term-care-homess/

Inspectorate in Scotland.[26]

So while susceptibility to illness was greatly increased, medical support was almost completely withdrawn, even GP support. Although staff members in nursing homes are medically qualified, this is not the case in the majority of care homes or among those providing community care. They are reliant upon primary care advice and intervention from their local GP. But the lockdown regime virtually removed GP support from care settings and the community and instead people were reliant on telephone consultations instead. There were zero visits.

Alzheimer's UK have many testimonies to illustrate just how devastating these actions were on their website, here is just one:

After 53 years of marriage, separation is very hard. Tony's wife, Sheila, was diagnosed with Alzheimer's disease in 2017 and currently lives in a care home. Following their enforced separation because of coronavirus, Tony shares how the lockdown has affected them, and a new poem.

> **"Before the coronavirus lockdown, I would make daily visits to the care home. Sheila always greeted me with a big smile, a kiss and a hug. I miss this very much. Blowing kisses via a video link is not the same."**
>
> **"I am losing some of the 'good days' left to us."**

The poem he was inspired to write for his wife, "Painted Lady Summer – By Tony Ward", is for public view on the Alzheimer's UK website and tells a sad yet beautiful tale.

"Between May and September 2019, over 10 million Painted Lady butterflies migrated from North Africa to Northern Europe – a once in a decade phenomenon."

Gavin Terry, head of policy at Alzheimer's Society, said that isolation can be devastating as family members and friends often play a crucial role in maintaining the health of people with dementia by bringing them meals, taking them out regularly to exercise and keeping people socially engaged. Withdrawing this support can cause people to rapidly go downhill, he said. **"We're hearing that some people are 'just giving up' or 'switching off' and not eating or drinking,"** he said.

---

[26] https://news.knowledia.com/CA/en/articles/isolated-uk-care-home-residents-fading-away-say-staff-and-families-fadb09a57eeb438bf1a4b8e87fc6eb8dfe385504

The article on Friday 5th June in The Guardian Online headlined: **"Extra 10,000 dementia deaths in England and Wales in April"** also stated:

> "Aside from coronavirus, in April there were a further 9,429 deaths from dementia and Alzheimer's disease alone in England and 462 in Wales. That number is 83% higher than usual in England, and 54% higher in Wales."

Clearly there was much concern about the policies being forced upon them.

May 7th 2020, in response to Boris Johnson's comment on the 6th May when he said he **"bitterly regrets"** the coronavirus crisis in care homes – and the government was **"working very hard"** to tackle it, Gavin Terry stated:

> "We haven't seen any evidence to suggest that deaths in care homes are slowing down, and any other implication would be dangerously complacent. In the past month, we know that the number of people who have died in care homes is twice the average; in the last week alone we saw the death rate rise by 30%. And it is not only deaths due to coronavirus that we fear - we are concerned there will be a sharp rise in deaths due to dementia, not least because of the impact of isolation, when the full figures are known."

People with dementia, who make up about two-thirds of the long-term care population, are particularly vulnerable. Many need partial or full feeding assistance, which takes time that staff don't always have. Changes in routine, such as being confined to their rooms because of an outbreak, often cause confusion and worsen symptoms. Two-and-a-half months after restrictions were put in place, family members and seniors advocates say there have been preventable deaths from dehydration and other residents are wasting away without the help of relatives and private caregivers they relied on at mealtimes. The loss of extra assistance comes as many facilities struggle with severe staffing shortages.

William Laing, the author of the new analysis on excess deaths among care home residents, said their treatment was **"a scandal which is just emerging."** He said he believed a series of failings were behind the high number of excess deaths:

> "At the peak of the crisis, there were widespread reports of normal medical support simply being removed from care homes," he said. "Ambulances would not turn up to take emergencies to hospital, since capacity had to be kept clear for Covid cases."

> Martin Green, chief executive of Care England, has commented, "the true scale of the coronavirus crisis 'burning through' care homes may never be known". He said in a scathing attack on the government's "herd immunity" policy: "I saw letters from GPs sent to care homes saying 'we will not be doing consultations, we will not be sending people to hospital'. I think there's a real issue that lots of people just were denied access to hospital."[27]

If the intention was to protect the most vulnerable, it is ludicrous to imagine that the cumulative effect of these policies didn't lead to early mortality among the most vulnerable. The lockdown regime was utterly devastating to the health of the very demographic it was supposedly designed to "keep safe".

I know of one lady who could not see her husband for the last week of his life because he was isolated in a "care home". They had been married for 67 years.

Hospital deaths

Regular rules and best practices for treating respiratory and influenza-type diseases ceased to be applied because of COVID-19 and instead new protocols were implemented with the focus being on minimising the spread of the virus rather than the best interests of the patient. One of these was the routine use of ventilation for suspected COVID patients and this was heavily promoted in the media and the supposed shortage of ventilators widely publicised. What was not publicised, however, was that this is an incredibly invasive and often deadly procedure involving a highly toxic cocktail of drugs and other interventions and that this was not the

---

[27] https://freedomnews.org.uk/care-homes-englands-culling-fields/

usual treatment method for patients presenting with symptoms of respiratory distress. A subsequent study in New York found that 80% of those ventilated died when ordinarily a death rate of 20% would have been expected.

Another protocol for treating COVID-19 featured in The Lancet and touted as the 'model treatment':

Here, the 50-year-old patient was given high doses of cortisone; methylprednisolone 600mg; moxifloxacin, a very strong antibiotic; a DNA gyrase inhibitor; Lopinavir and Ritonavir (both protease inhibitors from AIDS treatments); and finally at the end another broad-spectrum antibiotic. This would be a highly toxic mix with interferons with immunosuppressive effects.

The patient, who was not in a risk group, unsurprisingly died.

Erin Marie Olszewski, a frontline nurse in New York reported publicly on this, going as far as saying she felt that these patients were being 'murdered' by a general lack of care, over vigorous diagnosing of COVID-19 and the ventilation used to treat them. Her story very much aligned with that of other doctors and nurses in the UK who have come forward or posted to social media, and who confirmed some of the worst aspects of these new protocols that were causing avoidable deaths. She went on to write a book about her experience in hospital during the crisis: *Undercover Epicenter Nurse: How Fraud, Negligence, and Greed Led to Unnecessary Deaths at Elmhurst Hospital*. This gives us a good insight into her experience.

> **"You've got doctors and nurses that, at that point, just didn't care because everybody was going to die anyway so what's the point? And then you have everybody on a ventilator. So, these patients can't even speak for themselves. They're at the hands of whoever is taking care of them."[28]**

Legally doctors are always on the safe side if they do 'everything' that is recommended. If the patient then dies, they have committed no error. If they haven't adhered to the recommended protocol and the patient dies, then they have a problem. Remember the first law, "do no harm". Combine this top-down, non-scientific approach, with the forced use of DNRs, financial incentives, and it is easy to see how the fear could have

---

[28] https://www.leanmachine.net.au/healthblog/frontline-nurse-speaks-out-about-lethal-protocols/

escalated and made the whole situation incalculably worse.

For anyone doubting this could happen, The British Medical Journal published a study where they estimated that iatrogenic death (death caused by medical examination or treatment) was the third leading cause of death in the US. There is no reason to think that this is not also the case in the UK especially with the over-action seen both in diagnosing and then in treating COVID-19 particularly in the beginning where the pressure to follow the standardised protocols will have be even greater.

Lastly, the following uncomfortable truth must also be considered. It has been previously and widely alleged in the media that NHS doctors have been prematurely ending the lives of thousands of elderly hospital patients because they are either difficult to manage or to free up beds. In the current crisis, where beds were considered a particular premium and recovery from COVID-19 unlikely, just how many elderly patients, without a proper analysis of their condition and who could have lived longer, were placed on an 'assisted death pathway' rather than given routine care? We already know that to free up space in hospitals, elderly patients were discharged into care homes to effectively die.

Community deaths

Aside from receiving DNAR notices through the post, the most vulnerable in the community were also sent letters telling them to stay at home to "protect the NHS".

Not only did ambulance response times increase exponentially, access to hospital treatment was actively deterred and community healthcare and GP support was withheld. Just like in care homes people had to get used to telephone consultations instead of examinations and home visits, hugely increasing the risk to the most vulnerable. Not to mention that for the same reasons as in care home facilities, those in the wider community who now found themselves isolated, terrified and without support, would have also had their susceptibility to illness immeasurably increased.

Being terrified of either contracting the virus or overwhelming the NHS had the effect of drastically reducing emergency admissions and in week 14 there were 100,000 less than in the same week the previous year! At a time when the increase in stress levels was huge, there was a 40% reduction in hospital attendances for heart attacks. People with acute need for cardiovascular treatment (including strokes) were not going to hospital as they otherwise would. There was also a substantial reduction in referrals for acute coronary syndrome as well as reports of people presenting late with complications due to having a heart attack, something that was never normally seen.

Around 170,000 people die every year from cardiovascular disease in the UK so a 40% reduction in callouts, along with substantially lower referrals would likely represent a huge proportion of these excess deaths.

Dr Sonya Babu-Narayan, Associate Medical Director of the British Heart Foundations, said:

"During the lockdown, A&E presentations for heart attacks and strokes dropped by more than half. This resulted in a huge increase of deaths in the home."

Professor Stephen Westaby (a leading heart surgeon) stated:

"We could see thousands of deaths from heart disease and cancer over the next six months. Their families will never forget this. Neither China nor Italy stopped treating these conditions despite the chaos there earlier this year. It's bizarre."

Conclusions

The evidence is clear that the lockdown has caused, and will continue to cause, ill health and death. If the response to a public health crisis is to withdraw healthcare from those who need it the most, a spike in mortality is the only possible outcome. Not only are those affected by the disease more likely to succumb to it, but increased mortality from every other comorbidity is hard wired into that lockdown policy.

Rather than a virus that had long been present, it is these lockdown measures that would account for the strong correlation between the imposition of healthcare-limiting lockdowns and sharp increases in mortality.

From Professor Denis Rancourt:

"Immediately, as soon as the pandemic was declared, no matter where you were on the planet, synchronously everyone at the same time had the start of that very large sharp peak that was the extra number of large deaths. So what I concluded in my paper that this peak is not natural. A peak like this has never been seen for any of these respiratory viruses. It's not natural for the following reasons:

It's too narrow. A viral infection of this type that normally spreads in a society will never be that narrow. You always get these broader peaks. So it's too narrow to be a natural peak and it occurred synchronously everywhere at the same time, which is crazy. It can't be an accident. And it is happening too late in the season. There has never been, in the recorded history of mortality, a sharp peak like this, this late in the winter season anywhere at any time. So it's a completely artificially created situation where immune vulnerable people, their deaths were accelerated by what we did to them. And what did we do to them? We isolated them from their families. We closed them into institutions. We closed the doors of the institutions. We didn't let the air come out. The air was filled with the aerosol particles containing the virus and we infected them all by closing them in and stressing them more than they would be normally because they were isolated, they weren't cared for as well and their family couldn't see them and they were frightened by the fact that they were hearing about this horrible pandemic. Now that kind of psychological stress is known scientifically to be a major cause of faulty immune responses and causing other diseases as well. So you don't do that and they did it."

And so I believe that's the mechanism by which they accelerated the rate of death of immune-deficient fragile people who would have died in the many weeks and months later, eventually in a natural way but instead they accelerated their deaths by doing this. This could be confirmed if the average death rate falls in the coming months, which could show many people died before their time. (Actually happening now as I am writing this.)

UK Column

Here are a couple of graphs from the UK Column team. They have been actively getting out real news and exposing a National and Global agenda for over a decade. I have had the pleasure of holding events with them and exchanging information and can say they are easily the best and most thorough research team in the UK. They have a small team of researchers doing deep investigations that go way beyond where the mainstream ends up. They have made connections for many years with the banking system, child abuse, wars of terror, the mess in the Middle East, sustainable development and climate madness, loss of common law and the web of control that has taken over councils all over the UK and in NGOs and more, which leads people to believe they can **"lead beyond authority"**.

The article, **"The NHS Common Purpose: Towards A Million Change Agents"**, gives us a deep insight in the "change" that is taking place right throughout society.[29]

One example of massive "change" in the NHS is the massive reduction in beds over the last twenty years. Every winter for as long as I can remember we see headlines of the NHS being over-stretched and with a growing population we have seen a reduction in beds of about 77,000, approximately 30%.

---

[29] https://www.ukcolumn.org/article/nhs-common-purpose-towards-million-change-agents

Annual number of hospital beds in the United Kingdom from 2000-2019[30]

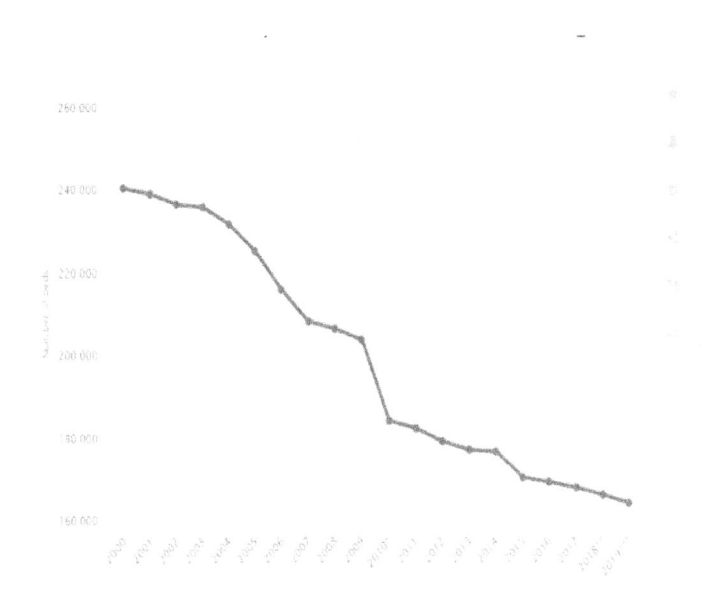

So here we have a clear agenda to massively reduce capacity of the NHS when they have openly been struggling for many years during the winter months. The NHS is ALWAYS under pressure. This cannot simply be put down to efficiency. This is an organised, conscious agenda to put massive pressure on the NHS. The unused Nightingale Hospitals should never have been needed, not that they were needed in reality anyway, but it did add to the show of fear and being overawed.

The only question people should be asking here is, "why the massive reduction with a growing population and an NHS already under pressure?" After all, this whole show was about "protecting the NHS".

The following graph put together by UK Column News show an eight-year cycle of deaths. Notice the large spike just after lockdown happened was later than in previous years and that there was the usual normal winter spike just before. Why the extra spike? Well, going from the previous information this certainly backs up the idea that this massive sharp rise in excess deaths was not a natural phenomenon and that the lockdown was in some way involved, if not a "novel new virus".

---

[30] Source – statista.com

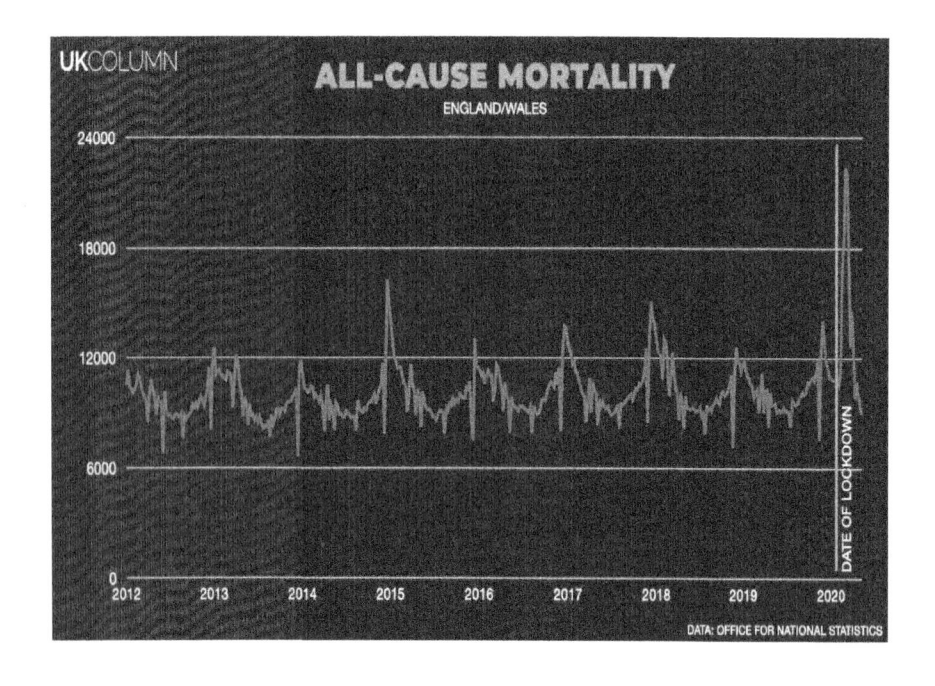

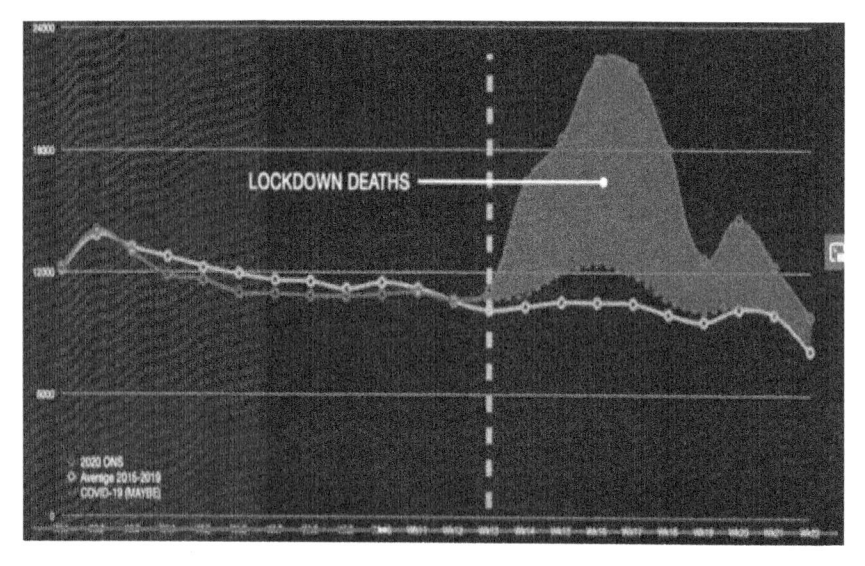

![All-cause mortality graph England/Wales 2012-2020 from UK Column, showing date of lockdown]

![Lockdown deaths graph comparing 2020 ONS, Average 2015-2019, and COVID-19 (MAYBE)]

The previous graph from the UK Column shows how the huge spike in deaths happened after the lockdown. With official information stating that maybe up to 30% of deaths were not "COVID-19" related, the UK Column took the Italian figure of 88% being only related to but not caused by COVID-19 and this shows what possibly may be a more accurate figure. Bear in mind this is a graph based on what came out of Italy and cannot be said to be totally correct but given all what we know about the lockdown protocols and who died in the UK, we can assume it cannot be far from correct.

The ONS stated:

> **"Of the deaths involving COVID-19 that occurred in England and Wales in March to May 2020, there was at least one pre-existing condition in 90.9% of cases; this is a similar level to that shown in March and April 2020."**

Conditions such as ischaemic heart disease, chronic pulmonary disease, diabetes, chronic kidney disease, chronic neurological disorder, dementia, asthma, rheumatological disorder, learning disability or autism and receiving treatment for mental health conditions.

So how do we know if the "virus" was increasing the mortality of already ill people or the government protocols and NHS treatment? The answer is, we don't until a full, open investigation is done but with the evidence at hand it does seem these mass extra deaths were due to political and medical decisions. It was well reported that medical staff were being gagged about talking about COVID-19 deaths and protocols. What is there to hide?

So going off the information on the graph, instead of showing a wave and onslaught of "COVID-19" deaths we may have just had a light ripple. What must be understood when testing positive for the SARS-CoV-2 is that dying "with" does not mean dying "from". Remember we also established the test only looks for part of the genetic sequence of the alleged virus; it is known not to be accurate, and at best only shows presence and in no way shows if it had anything at all to do with causing the disease in the first place, or whether it was one of many causal factors or just debris from the disease. No one has yet done any science to show this "novel virus" is causing disease.

It was well known doctors were putting down "COVID-19" as cause of death even if it was just suspected. I personally know of one lady who lost an elderly relative early in the crisis who tested negative but was still put down as a "COVID-19" death. So if someone died of cancer but at death tested positive it was allowed to be also counted as a "COVID-19" death.

Or even if someone died of a long-term illness or even old age – we all die eventually. If "COVID-19" was symptomatically there then it was also put on the death certificate, artificially inflating COVID-19 deaths. I also know of one lady who had at least fifteen years of illness and breathing issues, wheelchair bound and other health issues and in her seventies and died of "COVID".

Let's be clear, one of the symptoms of dying, in fact the main and last symptom, is lack of breath. But 24 hours a day we got the ever increasing death rate of "COVID-19" ripping through society via government updates and shamelessly repeated through the mainstream media. And again, nothing said about boosting your immune system with fresh air, supplements, sunlight and deep breathing. Just run and hide and hope and pray it doesn't get you and your loved ones.

FEAR FEAR FEAR

Death from anxiety

Imagine for a moment an individual who suffers from anxiety, watches all the media and government updates on the "deadly virus", believes everything and goes into total fear, fight or flight, except there is nothing to fight and nowhere to run to. It is quite possible for a person suffering from anxiety that he/she could go into a panic state and it affects their breathing. *I've got it, I'm sure I've got it.* Then imagine calling an ambulance; they arrive ready for the next virus case, your breathing is difficult and they rush you straight to the "COVID ward". You arrive into the "war zone"; people with masks on everywhere ready to deal with another victim and your anxiety now goes through the roof. *Am I gonna survive?* is in your head. You are put on the protocols in place and they see your breathing is getting worse and not better; this in turn makes your stress worse and breathing even more difficult. You are then put on a ventilator and after that it is in the hands of God.

This is a scenario that is possible and caused by anxiety and stress alone, brought on by the politicians, experts and media constantly telling us we need to be afraid of this invisible enemy coming to get us all. No virus needed in this scenario to explain the symptoms.

Obviously I am not trying to say anxiety = COVID-19 in all cases, but as we have seen in this book there are nearly always many factors to consider in an illness situation, getting run over by a bus aside, and in the main the medical doctors are solely obsessed in just looking at the symptoms and believing it is as simple as a viral attack.

Getting to the truth would mean an individual investigation into all "COVID deaths"; that obviously would be very difficult to do and would still not give us an absolute truth about each death but it may rule out the theory that there is one single cause when there is a sharp rise in the average death rate. What is clearly known about fear and anxiety is that it lowers what they call the immune system response. Evolution has created a fight-or-flight reaction to danger; when that happens our energy goes away from our inner body, where our main cleansing happens, and to the outer muscles so we can use the extra energy to escape the danger. This means normal immune function is almost stopped to get us out of danger but returns quickly after the danger has been evaded without much effect on the body. This should be a short-lived scenario but when we are put under permanent, chronic stress then we go into a permanent low level of fight or flight and the extra anxiety restricts our breathing as we can't relax. Over time this will seriously affect your health, especially if you are already have ongoing issues. It's not rocket science, really, just simple common sense.

Sweden

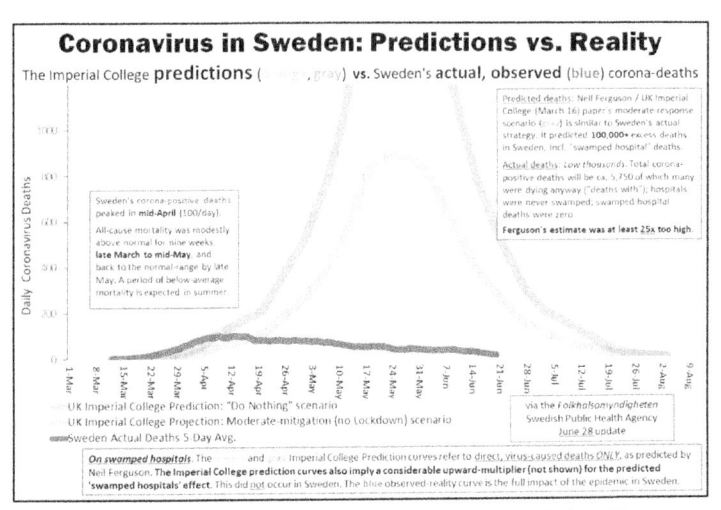

Coronavirus in Sweden: Predictions vs. Reality

The Imperial College **predictions** (gray) vs. Sweden's actual, observed (blue) corona-deaths

Predicted deaths: Neil Ferguson / UK Imperial College (March 16) paper's moderate-response scenario is similar to Sweden's actual strategy. It predicted 100,000+ excess deaths in Sweden, incl. "swamped hospital" deaths.

Actual deaths: Low thousands. Total corona-positive deaths will be ca. 5,750 of which many were dying anyway ("deaths with"); hospitals were never swamped; swamped hospital deaths were zero.

Ferguson's estimate was at least 25x too high.

Sweden's corona-positive deaths peaked in mid-April (100/day).
All-cause mortality was modestly above normal for nine weeks, late March to mid-May, and back to the normal-range by late May. A period of below-average mortality is expected in summer.

— UK Imperial College Prediction: "Do Nothing" scenario
— UK Imperial College Projection: Moderate-mitigation (no Lockdown) scenario
— Sweden Actual Deaths 5-Day Avg.

via the *Folkhälsomyndigheten* Swedish Public Health Agency June 28 update

On swamped hospitals: The and Imperial College Prediction curves refer to direct, virus-caused deaths ONLY, as predicted by Neil Ferguson. The Imperial College prediction curves also imply a considerable upward-multiplier (not shown) for the predicted 'swamped hospitals' effect. This did not occur in Sweden. The blue observed-reality curve is the full impact of the epidemic in Sweden.

https://swprs.files.wordpress.com/2020/07/sweden-projection-reality-june-28.png

Above is a graph showing what would have happened in Sweden going off Neil Ferguson's "expert" method in predicting disease patterns. As was well reported, Sweden was one of those countries that did not go into lockdown. The public health authority banned gatherings over 50 people, closed high schools and universities, and advised people to keep a safe distance. Basically let them get on with life and told them to use their own common sense. We had the whole world governments and media announcing their arrogance around this "deadly virus" and people sat back and looked for the coming disaster, very similar to what happened in Leicester in 1885.

What happened? We'll let the data tell us.

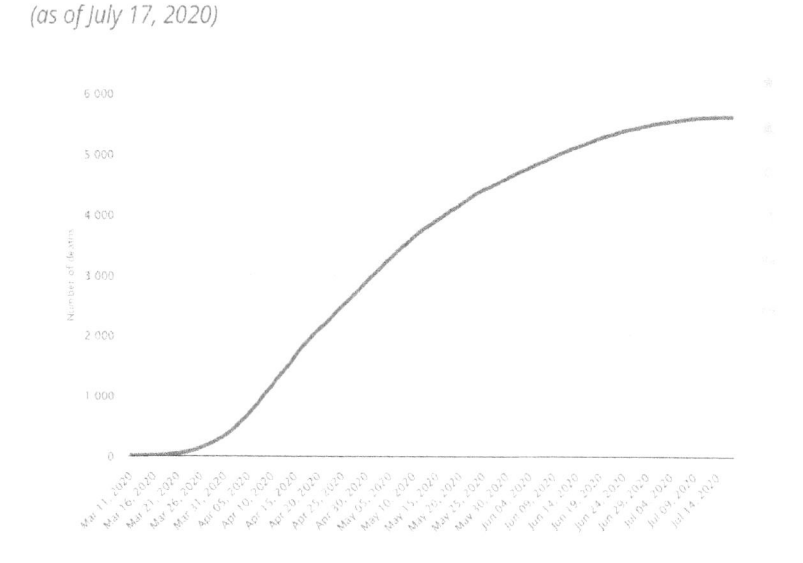

(as of July 17, 2020)

Graph of number of "COVID-19" deaths in Sweden in 2020 by age groups as of 17th July.

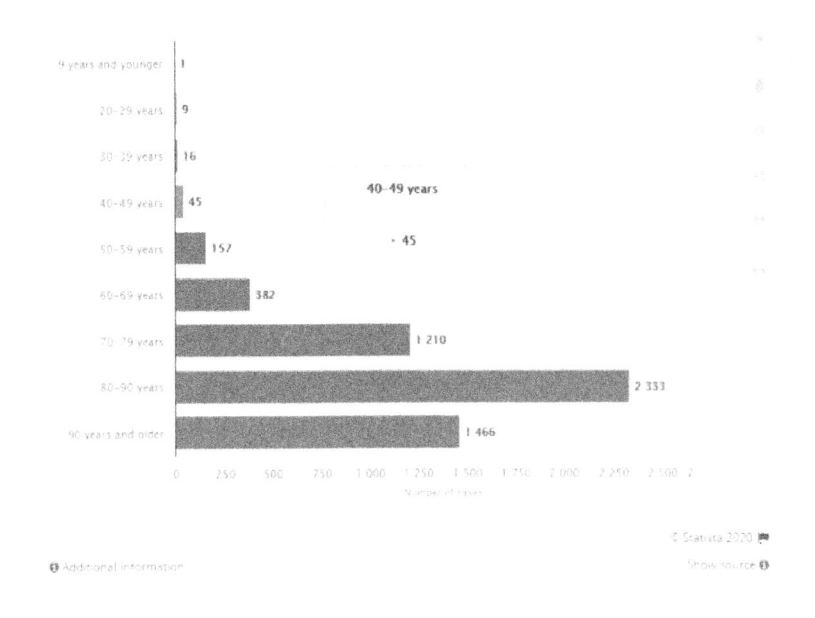

Age group	Number of cases
9 years and younger	1
20-29 years	9
30-39 years	16
40-49 years	45
50-59 years	157
60-69 years	382
70-79 years	1 210
80-90 years	2 333
90 years and older	1 466

© Statista 2020

The first thing to notice is that the "COVID-19" death rate followed a similar pattern to the UK and in fact, a smaller death rate per million, so from that, it is clear Sweden was less affected despite not going into lockdown. Sweden did, though, still have a fairly high death rate from "COVID-19". The vast majority of deaths occurred in the people 70 years and above and in fact, for the 60s and under it was quite a non-event. What was significant, though, was that on 31st March Sweden introduced its care home policies, including a ban on visits.

As reported by the BBC, 19th May 2020:

Coronavirus: What's going wrong in Sweden's care homes?

"Many care home workers were coming forward to criticise regional healthcare authorities for protocols which they say discourage care home workers from sending residents into hospital, and prevent care home and nursing staff from administering oxygen without a doctor's approval, either as part of acute or palliative (end-of-life) services.

"They told us that we shouldn't send anyone to the hospital, even if they may be 65 and have many years to live. We were told not to send them in," says Latifa Löfvenberg, a nurse who worked in several care homes around Gävle, north of Stockholm, at the beginning of the pandemic.

"Some can have a lot of years left to live with loved ones, but they don't have the chance... because they never make it to the hospital," she says. "They suffocate to death. And it's a lot of panic and it's very hard to just stand by and watch."

Mikael Fjällid, a Swedish private consultant in anaesthetics and intensive care, says he believes **"a lot of lives"** could have been saved if more patients had been able to access hospital treatment, or if care home workers were given increased responsibilities to administer oxygen themselves, instead of waiting for specialist COVID-19 response teams or paramedics.

So it is clear that what went wrong in Sweden nearly all took place in care homes and with the elderly in the community despite the Swedish authorities saying that shielding risk groups was its priority.

"We did not manage to protect the most vulnerable people, the most elderly, despite our best intentions."

– Prime Minister Stefan Löfven

It is very clear from the data that if it wasn't for the massive mistakes in policy set out to protect the vulnerable which resulted in a major cause of many premature deaths of those very same people, then Sweden would have breezed through all this and all with no lockdown, no masks and no economic suicide. Other data has shown that the number of "COVID" deaths is about the same as the excess deaths for that period, excess deaths that can be blamed on the policies alone.

Why is this obvious fact being ignored by world governments and medical authorities who are constantly reminding us we are all doomed and there is nothing we can do except to wait for a vaccine? By now it should be very clear that at the least something is very, very, wrong.

Japan

Japan, like Sweden did not introduce any hard lockdown at all or even go with the mass testing. They did order a state of emergency and people and non-essential businesses were asked to stay at home but there were no penalties for not doing so. Allegedly, Japan has more elderly people per capita than anywhere else in the world, and very densely populated cities. This, you would expect be the perfect breeding ground for this "deadly virus". When looking at the data, though, it seems hardly anything at all has happened. In fact, if you look at the cases and deaths from "COVID" it hasn't seemed to raise the average deaths expected at all. Remember, an average is just that and slightly above and below is also perfectly normal; only a real large spike would suggest something out of the normal which has not happened. Bear in mind, the testing is totally unreliable and again, dying "with" does not mean dying "of" and perfectly healthy people can test positive and ill people can test negative, so the only data that means anything is the death rate.

Total Coronavirus Deaths in Japan

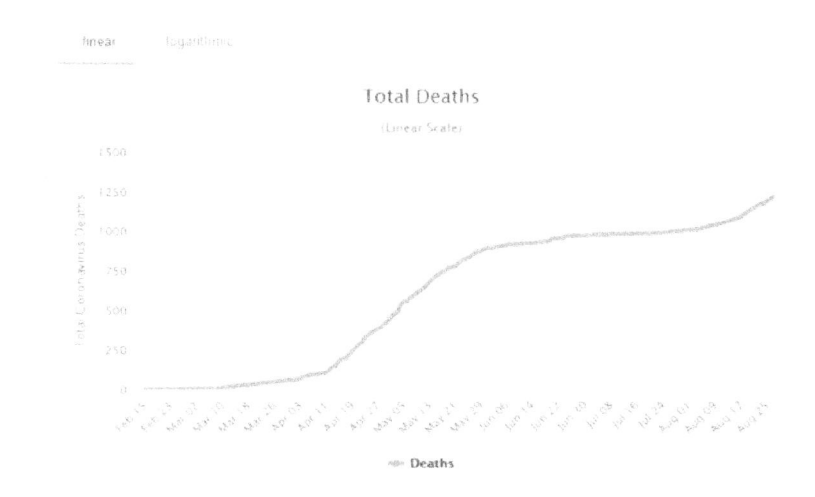

With a population of around 126 million and around 38 million in Tokyo alone, you would certainly think any "deadly virus" would have a field day especially within the elderly population. But it hasn't and in fact, if it wasn't for the testing then it could easily be said nothing at all out of the normal has happened. This, like Sweden, is a problem for the people pushing the official narrative and it will be interesting to see what happens in the near future.

Will they ramp up testing and sell the idea of chaos and an involvement in the global pandemic with just positive cases alone? Will they then lead into a lockdown which will then lead to mass deaths and a sharp rise in excess deaths which can then be blamed on the "deadly virus"? I don't know, but what is for sure is Japan, like Sweden, is a huge problem for those wanting to sell the "deadly virus" story and the idea that all we can do is lockdown and close society. The following example of Peru, with one of the earliest and strictest of lockdowns, is a great example to compare the two outcomes.

Peru

Peru is an interesting case for me as I have spent about two years there living in Lima and the Amazon capital Iquitos, two of the most affected areas. I know the living conditions and the environment and it is easy for me to see why the deaths occurred only after lockdown.

When the lockdown began men were allowed out only twice a week to shop and exercise; women also twice a week but on separate days with compulsory mask wearing at all times outdoors. With many people living in small apartment rooms, many with shared bathrooms, few of the large population of Lima having outside garden space, still a hot time of the year, it is not difficult to see that this could have an adverse effect on health. In Iquitos with the all-year-round hot and humid climate, with again, many people living in houses with no gardens (surprisingly, in a large jungle town but that is how it is structured) and very unsanitary conditions in Belen by the river with, again, mask use, then why would it be a surprise people were getting ill? Add to this a tendency for Latin people to be easily pushed into "group think" and "herd mentality", something the politicians use to great effect during elections, then this was always a recipe for fear and conditions creating a public health disaster.

As you can see according to worldometers there was not one single death from "COVID-19" before the lockdown. I know we still have the problem of what actually is a "COVID death" but from their viewpoint nothing happened before lockdown.

Total Coronavirus Deaths in Peru

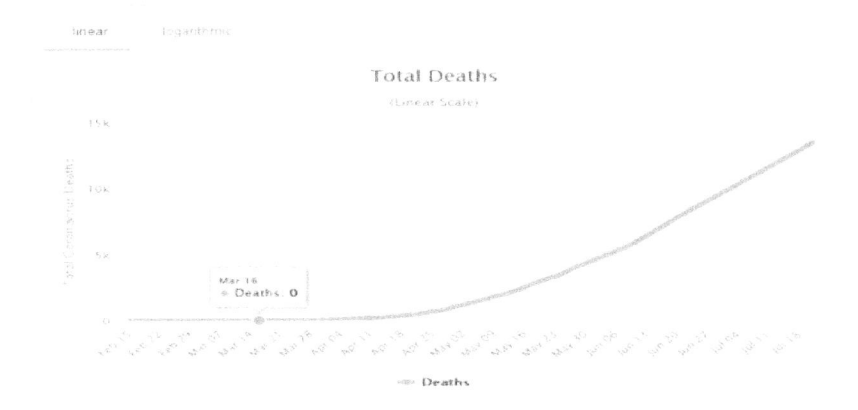

Graph from worldometers

USA

I could easily do a long chapter on the USA but why? It's all Dr Fauci-run and his connection to Bill Gates is very clear. He was on the Leadership Council for this Gates Vaccine initiative, enough said.

From the CDC 21/2/21:

Comorbidities and other conditions

Table 3 shows the types of health conditions and contributing causes mentioned in conjunction with deaths involving coronavirus disease 2019 (COVID-19). The number of deaths that mention one or more of the conditions indicated is shown for all deaths involving COVID-19 and by age groups. For 6% of these deaths, COVID-19 was the only cause mentioned on the death certificate. For deaths with conditions or causes in addition to COVID-19, on average, there were 3.8 additional conditions or causes per death.

2020/2021	All Sexes	0-17 years	204
2020/2021	All Sexes	18-29 years	1,684
2020/2021	All Sexes	30-39 years	5,030
2020/2021	All Sexes	40-49 years	13,482
2020/2021	All Sexes	50-64 years	70,160
2020/2021	All Sexes	65-74 years	103,451
2020/2021	All Sexes	75-84 years	133,557
2020/2021	All Sexes	85 years and over	151,344
2020/2021	All Sexes	All Ages	478,912

Taken from the CDC website dated 24/2/21

So again, a very clear picture of people dying with many comorbidities and mainly aged. And remember again, the 6% who died with no known health issues were found positive with a completely meaningless test in diagnostic terms. The UK Column also reported the difference between lockdown states and non- or less-lockdown states and again, the lockdown states seemed to be worse affected.

Mask Madness – Mask Murder

On the 24th July 2020, just a couple of days after Michael Gove saying they were not going to mandate masks, the self-proclaimed "right and honourable" Mat Hancock announced: **"Face coverings to be mandatory in shops and supermarkets from 24 July"**.

The reason:

> **"the death rate of sales and retail assistants is 75% higher among men, and 60% higher among women than in the general population. So as we restore shopping, so we must keep our shopkeepers safe."**

This statement, though, did not come with any science to back it up. I guess we'll have to take their word for it, like when they said bus drivers are dropping like flies, and they said it so it has to be true. It should be clear by now that when they want to pass some legislation it doesn't matter at all that they haven't got any science to back it up, just pass the new rules and they'll make it up as they go along or find a study soon enough. Irrespective of whether there are another thousand studies that say the opposite, the only data they want is what backs up their story. Worth noting even the WHO had no studies to back up mask wearing and it does seem that the change was politically driven and not scientific.

Again, note how they play with our minds, something we will be going into more. They say no, then they do it anyway. This creates the confusion they want. In the height of the "pandemic" in the UK there were very few people locally here wearing masks despite many people dying. But when the government announced it was a new needed measure, even though deaths were falling rapidly, the people who before had no interest in mask wearing were now convinced, not by facts but by fear, that it was the best thing to do.

We now have society split into the socially responsible mask wearer and allegedly the arrogant and selfish non-mask-wearer. And with Police Chief Cressida Dick stating, **"My hope is that the vast majority of people will comply, and that people who are not complying will be shamed into complying or shamed to leave the store by the store keepers or by other members of the public,"** it became clear we were going to be played off on each other, more divide and conquer. This woman is a disgrace and should be fired on the spot and charged with inciting if not violence then at least unlawful harassment.

Many doctors have stated that masks cannot protect from virus penetration. **"It's like putting a chain mail fence up to protect from mosquitos."**

And as for the safety aspect, well, the UK Column News 12th August 2020 showed that there has been no government risk assessment at all. It doesn't take a rocket scientist to see that restricting your own breathing cannot be good for your health; you are limiting the amount of oxygen you can take in and not allowing all the waste air out so you breathe in your own waste. Clean air in, dirty air out, that is what your breathing is about, and forcing back in what has just come out as waste is pure madness and I'm gobsmacked at the number of people who have been taken in by this madness. As a friend told me, **"it's mandated self-harm"**.

It shows a lot about the level of evil controlling society, and sadly even more about the lack of critical thinking within society. It should be clear that mask wearing is a psychological exercise to take away our power, individualism and humanity. The long-term effect will not just be the breathing issues but the mental health problems caused, especially for the young ones. Imagine a baby seeing its parents most of the day as mask wearers; this will disconnect and confuse them and affect their psychological and emotional development. But one man's symbol of slavery can also be sold to another's as a symbol of their caring, selfless, virtuous nature. Belief does control perception.

If masks are safe why the exemptions? What does the mask symbolise to you?

Clean hands please

Again, do we really need a discussion of why it is bad to put toxic hand cleansers on your hands multiple times a day?

More madness, and remember the skin is the body's biggest detoxification area so it opens up to let things out; this means it is also open to things going in, and toxic hand sanitiser going in simply cannot be good. It would be easy to look up scientific data on this but come on, folks, if you need scientific data for this then there is no hope. Sure, public health measures and hygiene were some of the things that caused the massive drop in infectious disease BEFORE vaccines, as we have seen, but wash your hands after the toilet and after work with soap and water and I think you'll live a long life.

I work outside and sometimes away from towns in the country and I have my "pee bushes", where after I may blow my nose after then eat my butties – we don't say "sandwich" in Manchester – after working all day with dirty water, I'm still alive and I never get ill and I don't think I'm that special. We are creating a nation of nervous hypochondriacs who feel under threat all the time and it is going to end in a lot of mental illness and anxiety.

Summer on the beach

Here in Cornwall, South-West England, when lockdown finally broke and we got the much-needed tourist money people were very fearful of what may happen. Well, it turns out two million "infected" tourists from the UK "hotspots" packing the beaches and the small Cornish towns actually made us healthier than ever. Yes, they put our deaths below average even with the "deadly virus" being brought in from all round the country.

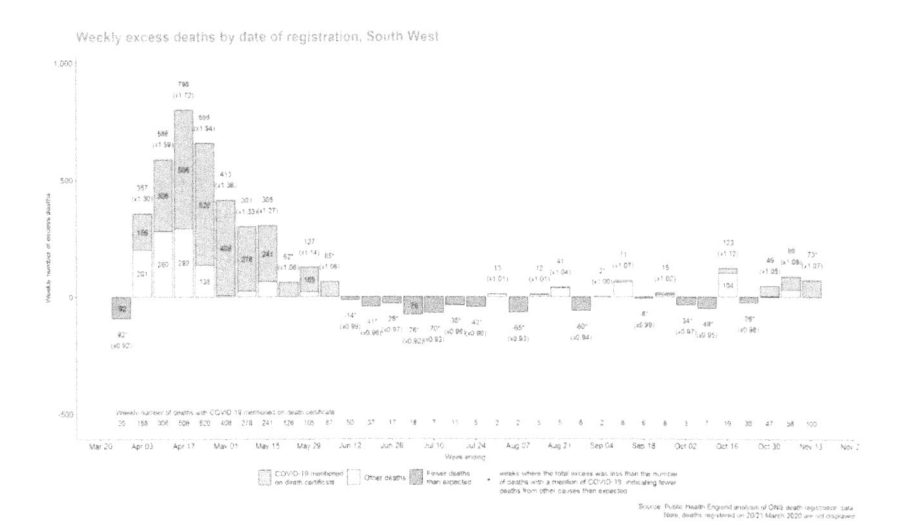

Weekly excess deaths by date of registration, South West

Notice the huge spike from the first lockdown and the drop way below average deaths in the busy summer, then the rise again as lockdown restrictions came back. Despite this data, Cornwall Council continue to push the closing of tourism until the "second wave" is under control. I have no idea what data they are looking at to make the statement that tourists are putting us at risk when it seems closing down Cornwall pushes the deaths up.

One healthcare assistant, Shelley Tasker from Treliske Hospital Cornwall, publicly resigned outside Truro Cathedral, a stunningly brave act from someone who could not live a lie. She stated she had basically been "twiddling her thumbs" through the "pandemic". Although slated in the local, mainstream and social media, all she stated was fact checked during a special interview with UK Column and shown to be correct. The crime she had committed was speaking the truth, a truth that affected the reputation of the worshipped NHS and their "hero" workers on "the front line", something the public could not allow.

This is a freedom of information reply from Royal Cornwall Hospitals where Shelley worked:

FOI Ref:11938

"From the 01st January 2020 to 24th November 2020 the Royal Cornwall Hospitals Trust had one deceased patient who tested positive for Covid 19 and had no pre-existing health conditions."

Again, this backs up what she had been saying and the fact that despite the packed Cornish summer, nothing actually really happened.

Freedom of Information Request Reference No: 01.FOI.20.014369

"How many police officers have died in the frontline in England, Scotland and Wales due to Coronavirus this year. This can be statistics provided in a table format and should include a category for ethnicity.

Please note that this response is in relation to MPS officers only, we do not hold data for the whole of the UK.

I have been advised that there have been no deaths of frontline officers in relation to the coronavirus."

So a long summer of protests in London with police charging and attacking peaceful, maskless protestors for freedom, and some not-so-peaceful "Black Lives Matter" protestors, and not one single officer dies of "COVID". Again, some "deadly virus".

SECOND WAVE OF MADNESS

Remember in "event 201" it was predicted that:

> **"65 million people dead in the first 18 months. The outbreak was small at first and initially seemed controllable but then it started spreading in densely crowded and impoverished neighbourhoods of mega cities. From that point on the spread of the disease was explosive. Within 6 months cases were occurring in nearly every country."**

Scarily accurate so far and from the beginning we have been warned of the second wave that is coming. So if it seems that the first wave was really mainly caused by the lockdown itself then what would this second and massively larger second wave be caused by?

Well it is very clear the lockdowns are not going away, except in Sweden where they were never present in the first place, don't let the world forget that one. They are here to stay whether they destroy life as we know it or not and regardless of the physical, emotional and economic harm they do.

In Victoria in Australia they have just announced a state of emergency could be in place for 18 months with just 430 "COVID" deaths to date and only 517 in the whole of Australia. Yes, and that 517 includes the state of Victoria. With people being dragged out of their cars after the windows were smashed by police just for not wanting to talk, it is very clear to state now that the government and police of Victoria are totally out of control, have lost the plot completely and are now a vicious police state that have turned on the people they are supposed to serve and protect.

It seems clear this is being driven by psychopathy and an insane, illogical belief that they are all gonna die unless the government take complete control. The police, repeating the line that the **"public must comply"** sends a shiver down my spine.

The second wave then will be created by months of people wearing masks and breathing in dirty air; by the time winter comes around when our body can struggle anyway due to the colder weather, less sunlight and less outdoor exercise, it is for sure that many people will suffer even worse than normal to cope and will become ill and probably have breathing issues.

Then we have what Matt Hancock announced in the UK as the biggest flu vaccine programme ever pushed on the population; a flu vaccine that has very little evidence, if any, of being effective anyway and is well known to have a side effect of the flu itself. I personally know people who have the flu vaccine and get the worst flu ever, yet the nurse tells them if it wasn't for the vaccine they would have probably died. No science to back that statement up but the people trust in them and they lap it up and queue up the next flu season to go through the whole thing again.

Then we have the normal flu season which can take tens of thousands of lives by itself. Can you see how all these things could be easily put down as the second wave? Add to that the same lockdown policies that will be repeated again despite massive failings the first time round and you can see globally where 65 million deaths could come from if the people go into total fear and compliance.

Peru has proven beyond doubt the damage of the lockdown and mask wearing. My sister-in-law now has "COVID", Feb 2021, except it's pneumonia and probably caused by the mask wearing. Her recovery plan, is antibiotics and stay in your room alone, isolated, without sunshine, until you are better. The debate is over, it is very clear; lockdown kills and as with Sweden (protect and shield policy aside), just getting on with life saves lives.

After a summer of empty hospitals but with the alert still high because of "cases", we come into late autumn/winter. In fact, if you even want to pursue their flawed science of "herd immunity" then summer would have been the perfect time to go for it as seems to be a time of the year when we could all come in contact due to our improved health during the summer months. This way deaths and illnesses would be low and we would all have "herd immunity" by winter when we know our systems are low and vulnerable. This would make sense and the coming winter disaster would be avoided and just maybe, our economy could survive. Why was this policy not pursued? Not that I believe in herd immunity but I am trying to use their understanding of disease to base an argument on their science. But as we have seen many times during this "crisis" the science keeps changing and now herd immunity is not possible as you can get "COVID" more than once.

Truth is, they have no plan, because the plan is the no-plan plan. The plan is to keep us controlled by fear with the new "cases" until winter is here. But they have lied, the curve has been flattened and there is no pressure on the NHS, in fact it's having a summer timeout as the hospitals are empty. The show is over and it's time to get back to living, or that's what the public thought.

We saw, as expected in the UK, the big flu vaccine programme and the lockdown measures being increased. Again, we see the rise in deaths occurring at a time when the normal "flu" season would start and yet as by magic, the "normal flu" seems to have disappeared and been replaced by "COVID".

"The second wave could kill 85,000", but it's safe to send your kids back to school.

> **"The evidence is overwhelming that it is in the interest of the wellbeing and the health of children, young people, pupils, to be back in school rather than missing out any more ... So, it is the healthy, safe thing to do."**
>
> – Boris Johnson

This is not politicians doing their best under difficult circumstances; this is very well thought out social destruction on a massive scale. So we have Johnson and Hancock still enforcing controlling laws, mandated masks in public, now being pushed in schools. It's safe but keep distancing, it's safe but the threat is still there, it's safe but many are gonna die in a second wave, it's safe but wear a mask, it's safe but wash your hands, it's safe but keep apart but at the same time go to school, it's safe but...

So now with schools closed down because apparently it wasn't safe after all, the deaths start to rise.

Whether you believe in the virus theory of disease or not is not relevant to the policy of destroying the ability for people to survive. To lock down the whole world and stop productivity is mass murder and I hope the people wake up to this fact sooner rather than later. Humanity needs to see that the governments are not our friends and instead of bringing in policies to avoid the coming disaster, they are actively bringing in policies to create hell on earth. This cannot be by accident, stupidity or ignorance.

Could it be the weak and vulnerable have died early last spring and now there were no more susceptible people left to be attacked in the summer, yet they keep preparing us for a second wave? We all know that every year winter flu-like illnesses are rife and the weak and old will die again. This will happen every year and there is nothing we can do about it. Wake up to the fact that death is as natural as life and life is for living.

I could put up many graphs and data to show what happened in winter in the UK but why? The same policies will give the same results.

"Insanity is doing the same thing over and over and expecting different results."

– Einstein

The two graphs here are taken from UK Column News as I know they take their national data from the ONS and their sources are always official. So again, we expected a rise in excess deaths due to the lockdown measures, especially in care homes. Remember, again, the most important aspects of health are clean air, sunshine, exercise, clean water and maybe most important, family and friends. Given that our tap water is polluted too then it could be easily said that to prepare for this "second wave" all the vital components of a healthy life were taken away and on top of that the constant fear, even an obvious supplement of vitamin D wasn't on the table. Again, no health measures, only fear measures. Then with the rollout of the experimental "COVID" vaccines, or gene therapy, for the aged, it didn't look good.

On the publishing of this book the UK Column have now created a special page on their website with the data direct from the MHRA yellow card scheme for Covid vaccine adverse reactions , on this day 27 may 2021 they have 235223 total reports with a total of 1180 fatalities. With the MHRA acknowledging they only ever get about 10% of severe adverse reaction reported again we are looking at the tip of a very big iceberg https://yellowcard.ukcolumn.org/yellow-card-reports.

OVER 80's COVID DEATHS

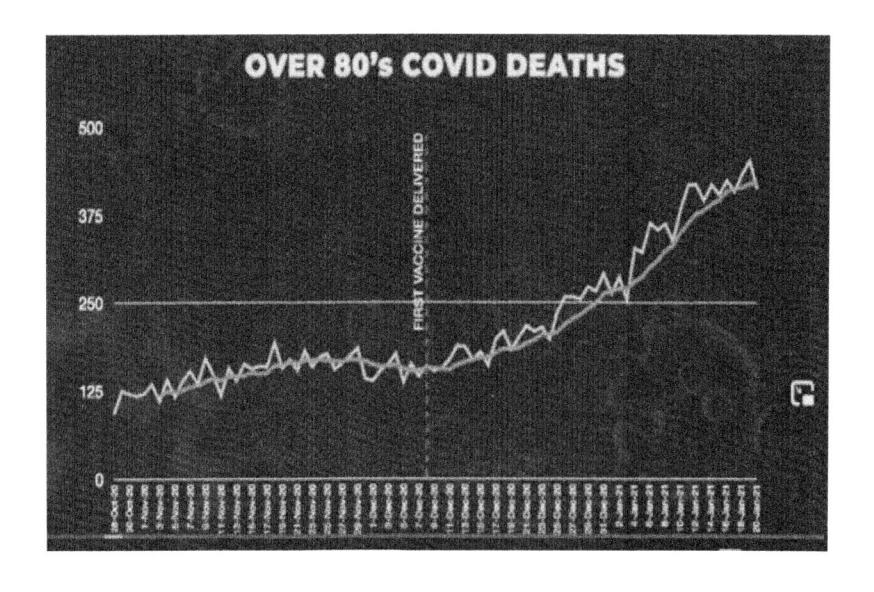

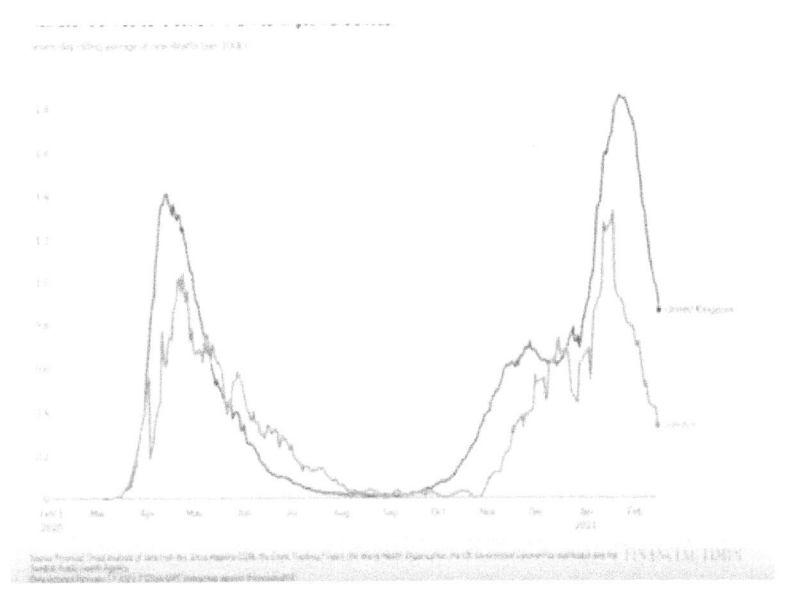

So the obvious correlation with the vaccine rollout and rise in over 80s deaths is clear. The connection does not mean cause and obviously other lockdown factors in care homes as mentioned above means this wasn't unexpected at all. This correlation alone should require the stopping of the experimental vaccine rollout until a full investigation is done, especially as the MHRA have already started reporting their expected

COVID vaccine deaths and adverse reactions and we are still only in February. This is not incompetence; it is murder, pure and simple. There is no way the self-proclaimed "leaders" and "experts" are so stupid they can't see this.

Again, to "save the NHS" during the "second wave" we seem the same tactics.

> **"Fury at 'do not resuscitate' notices given to Covid patients with learning disabilities"**
>
> – The Observer Online, Sat 13th Feb 2021

> **"People with learning disabilities have been given do not resuscitate orders during the second wave of the pandemic, in spite of widespread condemnation of the practice last year and an urgent investigation by the care watchdog.**
>
> **Mencap said it had received reports in January from people with learning disabilities that they had been told they would not be resuscitated if they were taken ill with Covid-19.**
>
> **The Care Quality Commission said in December that inappropriate Do Not Attempt Cardiopulmonary Resuscitation (DNACPR) notices had caused potentially avoidable deaths last year."**

So we have the aged again dying by the thousands and a clear and vicious attack on people with learning difficulties. This is Eugenics, pure and simple.

Then we look at what difference the lockdown made compared with non-lockdown Sweden and the pattern is the same, again, we have closed the country and wrecked the economy and lives of people and children's education for nothing. The full-year pattern of excess deaths in Sweden follows the UK yet their lives and economy and more importantly mental health have not been destroyed.

The last real question is, do the deaths add up to the worst "plague" since the great Spanish flu? This is what the public are being told but as usual, most people just read the big headlines, take that as truth and as we know the devil is always in the details.

As we have established, the only figure that can be relied upon is the deaths. How bad was this "pandemic"? The figure out for England and Wales for 2020 is 608,002 deaths. We are told the worst deaths since the "Great Spanish Flu" a century ago. Well, if you just take a simple number like that and blow it up in the mainstream media knowing that most people just read headlines then that is a very powerful figure.

An obvious thing to state would be the large population rise since those times so death rates give far more information, and also in 1976, the year of the great drought, some 599,000 people died in England and Wales, not too far off 2020 deaths and with a growing population, yet I remember that summer of water shortages and hot sun without a care in the world. Certainly I don't remember any government or media frenzy telling us to fear for our lives. I do though, remember lots of fun playing football in the park and Manchester United losing a dramatic FA Cup final.

2. Long-term trends in mortality

The charts below show the number of deaths and the crude death rate in different parts of the UK, in each year from 1961 to 2017.

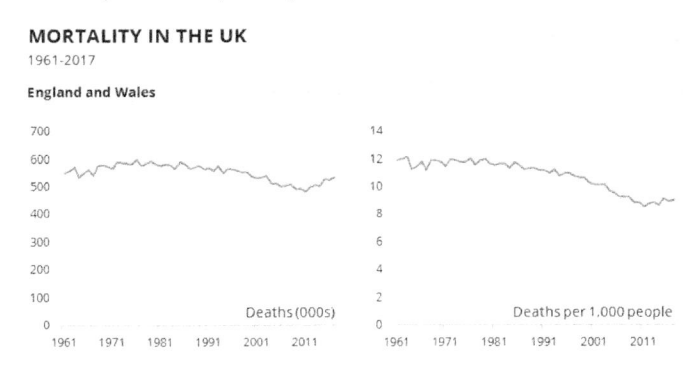

MORTALITY IN THE UK
1961-2017

England and Wales

House of Commons Library briefing paper, Number CBP8281, 14th Jan 2018

The number of deaths in the 60s and 70s age bracket were certainly high considering the lower population and the death rates were much higher, which gives a more accurate figure as it takes in population rises.

So if we go to the ONS data for the last thirty-one years, next on the page there were 14 years with a higher "crude mortality rate" for 2020 for England and Wales. For the "age-standardised mortality rate" which some would say gives a more accurate assessment of the factors there were 19 years with a higher rate. With 2020 having an age-standardised mortality rate of 1,043 per 100,000 and looking at the tables below, you can see it certainly has not been an exceptional year especially when comparing with the period between 1960-1980 when crude deaths rates were much higher. Coming out of normal "flu season" now, end of Feb, we would expect to see excess deaths go down as they normally do, only this time it will be the "lifesaving vaccine" that reduces the deaths and not the spring sunshine.

When you take off what must be, in my opinion, thousands if not tens of thousands of lockdown deaths from various factors as shown earlier, then the question must be asked. Has anything unusual actually happened at all?

Year	Number of deaths	Population (Thousands)	Crude mortality rate (per 100,000 population)	Age-standardised mortality rate (per 100,000 population)
2020	608,002	59,829	1,016.20	1,043.50
2019	530,841	59,440	893.1	925
2018	541,589	59,116	916.1	965.4
2017	533,253	58,745	907.7	965.3
2016	525,048	58,381	899.3	966.9
2015	529,655	57,885	915	993.2
2014	501,424	57,409	873.4	953
2013	506,790	56,948	889.9	985.9
2012	499,331	56,568	882.7	987.4
2011	484,367	56,171	862.3	978.6
2010	493,242	55,692	885.7	1,017.10
2009	491,348	55,235	889.6	1,033.80
2008	509,090	54,842	928.3	1,091.90

2007	504,052	54,387	926.8	1,091.80
2006	502,599	53,951	931.6	1,104.30
2005	512,993	53,575	957.5	1,143.80
2004	514,250	53,152	967.5	1,163.00
2003	539,151	52,863	1,019.90	1,232.10
2002	535,356	52,602	1,017.70	1,231.30
2001	532,498	52,360	1,017.00	1,236.20
2000	537,877	52,140	1,031.60	1,266.40
1999	553,532	51,933	1,065.80	1,320.20
1998	553,435	51,720	1,070.10	1,327.20
1997	558,052	51,560	1,082.30	1,350.80
1996	563,007	51,410	1,095.10	1,372.50
1995	565,902	51,272	1,103.70	1,392.00
1994	551,780	51,116	1,079.50	1,374.90
1993	578,512	50,986	1,134.70	1,453.40
1992	558,313	50,876	1,097.40	1,415.00
1991	570,044	50,748	1,123.30	1,464.30
1990	564,846	50,561	1,117.20	1,462.60

IT'S ALL A MIND GAME

Mindspace – influencing behaviour through public policy – extracts from the document:

> "Influencing people's behaviour is nothing new to Government, which has often used tools such as legislation, regulation or taxation to achieve desired policy outcomes. But many of the biggest policy challenges we are now facing –such as the increase in people with chronic health conditions –will only be resolved if we are successful in persuading people to change their behaviour, their lifestyles or their existing habits. Fortunately, over the last decade, our understanding of influences on behaviour has increased significantly and this points the way to new approaches and new solutions."

Why "social distancing" and not "physical distancing"?

> "Influencing behaviour is central to public policy. Recently, there have been major advances in understanding the influences on our behaviours, and government needs to take notice of them. This report aims to make that happen."

> "The vast majority of public policy aims to change or shape our behaviour. And policy-makers have many ways of doing so. Most obviously, they can use "hard "instruments such as legislation and regulation to compel us to act in certain ways. These approaches are often very effective, but are costly and inappropriate in many instances. So government often turns to less coercive, and sometimes very effective, measures, such as incentives (e.g. excise duty) and information provision (e.g. public health guidance) – as well as sophisticated communications techniques."

I recommend for everyone to watch on YouTube "The Century of the Self" by Adam Curtis. In it he shows how for over a century – actually a lot, lot longer – western governments, again really all governments, have been using their knowledge of psychology to control and guide public behaviour. Edward Bernays, nephew of Sigmund Freud, invented the public relations profession in the 1920s and was the first person to take Freud's ideas to manipulate the masses. He showed American corporations how they could make people want things they didn't need by systematically linking mass-produced goods to their unconscious desires. A very simplified understanding is that many people are driven by their fears and their desires. Ultimately our greatest desire is to freely express ourselves.

So given this knowledge and given that behaviour change is openly being used by the British politicians and the organisations and institutions that are running society, we really need to start to look at what the government want us to think and how they want us to behave. They don't even hide the fact.

A look into the "MINDSPACE" document should be followed by the "Behavioural Insights Team" also known as the "nudge unit".

On the GOV website it states: **"Behavioural Insights Team is now independent of the UK government"**, meaning it was part of the UK government before.

So, a look to the new website: https://www.bi.team/

> **"We apply behavioural insights to inform policy, improve public services and deliver positive results for people and communities."**

Remember earlier we showed that Dr Halpern is chief executive of the government-owned Behavioural Insights Team, known as the "nudge unit", and a member of Whitehall's Scientific Advisory Group for Emergencies (Sage) and also co-authored a government document titled "MINDSPACE". It is the SAGE team who it seems are running the show and giving the government the "best available science" which in turn is making the policies which are taking our freedoms away, destroying our economy and destroying our lives. So it is very clear that the government is using psychological techniques on the public. Why?

Well, as we will see next, at the foundation of behaviour is belief, and if you can control the beliefs of the population then you can easily control their behaviour.

Do you remember earlier the words of Boris Johnson after the ridiculous prediction of Neil Ferguson?

> **"This is the worst Public health crisis in a generation"** ... **"and I must level with you and the British public, more families, many more families, are going to lose loved ones before their time."**
>
> – Boris Johnson, 12th March 2020.

This is what started the biggest psychological experiment the UK has ever seen, but it was just a part of a bigger global experiment; only this experiment wasn't about testing theories, it was about putting them into practice.

"Options for increasing adherence to social distancing measures 22nd March 2020"[31] was prepared for the Scientific Advisory Group for Emergencies (SAGE). The paper was discussed at SAGE meeting 18 on 23rd March 2020. Extracts from document:

> "Perceived threat: A substantial number of people still do not feel sufficiently personally threatened; it could be that they are reassured by the low death rate in their demographic group(8), although levels of concern may be rising(9). Having a good understanding of the risk has been found to be positively associated with adoption of COVID-19 social distancing measures in Hong Kong (10). The perceived level of personal threat needs to be increased among those who are complacent, using hard-hitting emotional messaging. To be effective this must also empower people by making clear the actions they can take to reduce the threat)."
>
> "Use media to increase sense of personal threat."
>
> "There are nine broad ways of achieving behaviour change:

---
[31] https://assets.publishing.service.gov.uk/government/uploads/system/uploads/attachment_data/file/882722/25-options-for-increasing-adherence-to-social-distancing-measures-22032020.pdf

Education, Persuasion, Incentivisation, Coercion, Enablement, Training, Restriction, Environmental restructuring, and Modelling."

Whatever your opinion is on the illness or why people are dying, it is very clear that the government is manipulating people's perceptions to control behaviour; notice they even used the phrase **"Perceived threat"**, and as I confirm, my own local MP has no idea this is going on. Yes, it seems that MPs do not know about the open use of psychological techniques being used on the British population by members of the cabinet office to instil fear and control our beliefs so they can make it easier for their policies to be accepted, policies that, again, are destroying the country and people's lives.

In 2017 the WHO published a document: **"Best practice guidance // How to respond to vocal vaccine deniers in public."**

> "This guidance document provides basic broad principles for a spokesperson of any health authority on how to respond to vocal vaccine deniers. The suggestions are based on psychological research on persuasion, on research in public health, communication studies and on WHO risk communication guidelines."

> "Prepare three key messages. A person's working memory is responsible for storing visual and vocal in-formation and is strongly restricted in capacity. The audience will not be able to recall or even transfer the provided knowledge when confronted with too much information. Prepare three key messages you really want the public to know and remember."

> "Repeat your key messages as often as reasonably possible."

So the message is clear: the general public are stupid and childlike (my words), so keep it simple with no more than three messages.

> "Stay alert – control the virus – save lives."
>
> "Hands – face – space."

Welcome to the biggest psychological operation the world has ever seen.

With them clearly wanting to affect our perceptions, we will look into this very interesting subject.

Perception

Bruce Lipton in his book *The Biology of Belief* changed the way we look at what controls human behaviour at a cellular level and also at the full human level. He showed that life is really just an exchange of information from your inner world to the outer world and vice versa. That exchange of information creates movement and that movement is what we call life. So you have your individual self, a condensed energy field of unique information made up of all your perceptions and beliefs, some inherited and some taken on through experience, nature and nurture. Information comes in from the outside world whether it is sight, sound, food, energies and more. For life to happen, for movement or behaviour, the information has to mean something to the energy field of the individual and that meaning is based on the beliefs of that human. This belief does not have to be factual or even rational, it just is what you yourself believe to be true. Belief and therefore perception is a very individual thing.

Information comes in, or as Rupert Sheldrake says we **"clothe reality"** with our perceptions. Say, the sight of a spider; it connects to your belief system, so let's say spider means danger and fear – your perception of the situation is that you are in danger and therefore a fight or flight behaviour will kick in, with all the needed chemistry in the body kicking in too. But again, it doesn't mean the spider is danger and fear, just that this is what you believe it to be, which may be based on a childhood experience of seeing a family member running away from a spider. Another human, though, may see a spider, and that spider could mean a beautiful part of nature. Yes, some people actually love spiders. This would then create a different behaviour, maybe handling the spider, and that would, again, influence the chemistry of the body. This is a very simple example of how it is your belief that controls your biology and therefore behaviour.

A quote from former doctor Patrick Quanten:

> **"The senses open up the conscious mind. It is the information picked through the senses that will make us aware of the environment, of the reality, but seen in a specific way and that is the way the brain, the**

> nervous system, interprets the incoming information. The brain plays an important part in the conscious mind. It plays no part in the mind itself. The conscious mind works through the matter and is linked to the brain function; the mind is an energy field that just is. The conscious mind is intrinsically linked to an individual. The mind exists without a body."

So all behaviour is individual and based on the beliefs of the individual and these beliefs will control perception and behaviour. Biology, and therefore behaviour, is not controlled by genes as Bruce Lipton shown, but by beliefs. In experiments he took out the nucleus of cells and they carried on functioning as normal; if life was controlled by genes then the cells would have died but the cells carried on functioning as normal. Their lifespan was cut short as without genes they couldn't reproduce or replace any failing parts. It turned out the brain of our cells is the membrane, which has countless antennae for all the incoming information and the antennae were mainly tuning into energetic information. They, like us as a whole, are receivers and transmitters of information, so belief that genes control life was not true and life wasn't about having the good or bad fortune to be born with certain genes and an inability to change things.

It turned out genes produce proteins and those proteins are connected to certain cellular behaviour, but all the decision making is done through the brain of the cell, the membrane, where the senses are. We as human beings are made up of over 60 trillion cells and have one central brain that takes in all information from all the cells and coordinates the behaviour of the whole person. He also showed that any local behaviour in the body by certain cells can be overridden by the main man in charge, your brain, and becoming conscious of our own beliefs then, it seems it is ourselves who are in charge of our biology and therefore behaviour, and we are not just victims of a bad roll of the dice.

So knowing that the government have full knowledge of how this works and that for at least a century this knowledge has been used by governments and corporations to control behaviour and even sell products, the obvious question to ask is how many of your beliefs have been put into your mind by government?

The British Government are forever talking about "change" and "vision".

"Govern" = control. "Ment" comes from Latin, mind = mind control.

What change do they mean? What vision do they have for the country and its people? And how will they get from where they are now to that vision? Why do public servants believe they have a right to "change" behaviour to fulfil their "visions" when they are here to serve us and not the other way around? I think this is a very dangerous and sinister game to be playing, especially as the vast majority of people have no idea that there is a game being played. It is impossible to live in a free country if all your perceptions are being manipulated to pursue the hidden agenda of criminal politicians.

The name of this agenda is "agenda 21", now "agenda 30".

Did you know the United Nations have a plan for the whole of mankind and how we will live? This agenda is about total control from cradle to grave of every man, woman and animal of the planet, and the environmental "green movement" and "climate change" movement are fully involved in this, the majority unknowingly, changing our beliefs and therefore our perception of what is going on, on the planet, and this will influence how we behave. Driving an electric car, for example, or going vegan.

> **"Because of the sudden absence of traditional enemies, "new enemies must be identified."**
>
> **"In searching for a new enemy to unite us, we came up with the idea that pollution, the threat of global warming, water shortages, famine and the like would fit the bill... All these dangers are caused by human intervention, and it is only through changed attitudes and behaviour that they can be overcome. The real enemy then, is humanity itself."**
>
> – Book by The Club of Rome, 1991, *The First Global Revolution*

It is very clear there has been a massive worldwide psychological campaign going on for a long time, to convince mankind we are changing the climate of the planet and therefore putting humanity and the planet in danger. They, again, use science that omits many factors in the climate and weather, like that big yellow thing in the sky. Did you notice how "global warming" has changed to "climate change"?

Priming the mind for a future event, conscious or subconscious mind, meaning telling you or the use of subliminal messages is another tactic used.

Dancing nurses, anyone? Go to Vimeo – "Predictive Programming ~ The

2012 Olympics from the UNITED KINGDOM".[32]

Jeremy Hunt oversaw the 2012 London event and as of 29th Jan 2020 became Chair of the Health and Social Care Select Committee. Strange coincidence!

St. Corona is also the patron saint of epidemics.

Throughout maybe Feb and March 2020, after watching a programme on Netflix, the next recommended view offered automatically was a film "Contagion", or it may have been "Pandemic", one or the other. I have never watched programmes like these but for a few weeks it kept coming up for me to watch, nothing else.

I urge everyone to watch the video of the song "Where Are Ü Now" by Justin Bieber. A video aimed mainly at young children. In it, you will find many disturbing images of death, sex and drugs, even aliens and more, images so fast that you cannot consciously see any of them but if you go slow enough or freeze frame them all will be revealed, even stating "Bush did 9/11", though I personally don't think he has the brains to organise that one. But anyway, why would you put disturbing images in a video like that knowing young people would see it? Not all will be affected, I know, but as we know the subconscious controls most of our life it is very disturbing indeed.

So a lot of things we see may be there to expose stuff going on, or maybe to prime our minds. "The Hunger Games" films, for example. Are we being warned or primed? George Orwell and Aldous Huxley – were they whistle blowers or primers of our minds? I suppose it depends how you take the information on an individual level. I have found *1984* and *Brave New World* helpful for me to understand how we are being manipulated.

In many films you will see all aspects of an agenda, like in James Bond films, and in the Marvel series "Captain America: the Winter Soldier" is very revealing.

So we have this onslaught on our minds to control our behaviour. From birth we are actually the coming together of two "mind fields" – minds with beliefs holding them together. We then develop in the mother's womb, feeding off her emotions and reactions so we can have at least an idea of the world we are coming into. Then for the first 6/7 years we just absorb all the incoming information and also the reactions of Mother at

---

[32] https://vimeo.com/408121823?fbclid=IwAR2S9ziB-2MyysV43MyqQ6GDoOPdXnPkcMhHoYPq_vv9suvPPAld0nNKvQc

first and then the surrounding family. These first 6/7 years can then create a human being ready to start to live in the world he/she lives in, but it is only a perception of the world. It is not all the world and some of those perceptions will be valid and some not, but we will start to live our life through those beliefs that will create a perception of the world we live in.

This is the reason they want our children in school as soon as possible. Nothing to do with "helping mothers back to work"; we have been fooled into believing that being a full-time mother is not a job in itself so the state can get into the minds of our children, hence control their future perceptions and behaviour. Pure *Brave New World* social engineering massively helped by the far left and hijacked feminist movement who want to free women. Notice it doesn't seem to be about being free to be women, but about being free to compete with men. What on earth is wrong about a woman just being a woman? Men and women are different, physically but also emotionally; a lot of the differences may be small but we are different. Having equal opportunity is one thing but being the same is another.

So now we go through life and as we get older we may, if we are lucky, start to challenge our own beliefs and behaviour which in turn can cause turmoil, which is needed to break down false beliefs and open our minds to more possibilities. It seems the best way to do this is really to stop for a while; take a deep breath, and just stop believing in anything and take a look at your behaviour and reactions to life and situations and try to see honestly why you react and behave a certain way. Find out whether certain behaviour is beneficial or holding you back; be honest with your emotional connection to things and start to put back beliefs which you feel are worthy, truthful and beneficial to yourself as an individual. An old way to do it would be to imagine a needle in a haystack – very difficult to go looking for the needle, the best way would be to throw out what is not the needle, the hay, and eventually what is left must be the needle. If the needle is truth and the hay is non-truths then it may be a good place to start to throw beliefs away that are false, holding you back, and see what you have left.

Whatever you do, always try be conscious of what you are doing and this way you do not have to be a victim of your subconscious behaviour and can start living a life in control by being conscious of how you feel and behave and why.

The **"Coronavirus Act"** will be implemented by people based on their perceptions of what is going on and what they are observing. We know perceptions are just that and not absolute truth; we also know we have a government keen on using techniques to control our perceptions and therefore control our behaviour. When this has been done, all amounts of horrors are possible by people "believing" they are doing right.

> "The receptivity of the masses is very limited, their intelligence is small, but their power of forgetting is enormous. In consequence of these facts, all effective propaganda must be limited to a very few points and must harp on these in slogans until the last member of the public understands what you want him to understand by your slogan."
> – Adolf Hitler

STAY SAFE – CONTROL THE VIRUS – SAVE LIVES – BIG BROTHER LOVES YOU

Suffer Little Children

Dr Bruce Lipton when talking about the Romanian orphan children mentioned how many of them turned out autistic. He talked about how they were well nourished physically but were completely malnourished in terms of love, affection and physical touch. Remember we spoke earlier about how a child develops through experience and perceptions based on beliefs. It doesn't take much working out to see the effect on development when there is little physical love or touch.

Humans are social beings and we are meant to hug our kids and each other; it is part of our physical, emotional and social development. The governing bodies of this world have mandated behaviour through a belief of a disease that makes human beings enemies of each other, even a baby an enemy to its mother or a mother a danger to her baby.

There is already mass autism in the world, behaviour defined by lack of social skills, repetitive behaviours, speech and nonverbal communication. I know of the history of Dr Wakefield and how he was attacked for giving his own scientific opinion, one that wasn't wanted; whether there was truth in it or not didn't matter. The gut biome and cognitive connection, though, is well known to science yet he mentioned the V word and he was done for. I do though, know of non-vaccinated autistic children and when we look at the work of Dr Patrick Quanten on the formation of a human being, the issues involved become very clear.

I arranged a seminar where he took us through the whole development of a human being from conception to adulthood and it became very clear to me that from conception, even at conception, the perceptions and therefore behaviours of the child are being formed. If a mother and father conceive and have a belief that the world is a very harsh and unforgiving place then that is the information that will form the child. If then throughout pregnancy the mother still sees the world as this terrible stressful place then for the child, that is the world he/she is coming into.

In the early years of a child's life the importance of feeling safe is maybe top of the list and the importance of a close physical relationship with close family with freely given and accepted hugs and physical play is also needed to create security and also close bonds. Tickle games are what kids seem to thrive on. If for some reason a child has had a bad start to life physically and emotionally then it is important to help them realise that healthy loving affection is natural thing. Helping bring about a strong trusting bond between child and parents is essential.

Theraplay – Developed in the USA in the 1980s by Phyllis Booth, a scientist, it has become increasingly recognised as highly beneficial in supporting attachment difficulties with parents and children.

The Theraplay Institute

"Theraplay is a dyadic child and family therapy that has been recognized by the Association of Play Therapy as one of seven seminal psychotherapies for children. Developed over 50 years ago, and practiced around the world, Theraplay was developed for any professional working to support healthy child/caregiver attachment. Strong attachment between the child and the important adults in their life has long been believed to be the basis of lifelong good mental health as well as the mainstay of resilience in the face of adversity. Modern brain research and the field of neuroscience have shown that attachment is the way in which children come to understand, trust and thrive in their world."

Core Concepts

"Theraplay uses practitioner guidance to create playful and caring

child-adult interactions that foster joyful shared experiences. These activities build attunement and understanding of each other – replicating early relationship experiences that are proven to lead to secure attachment. The interactions are personal, physical and fun – a natural way for everyone to experience the healing power of being together."

"With the support of the Theraplay practitioner, parents learn to play with their child in a way that establishes felt safety, increases social engagement, expands arousal regulation, and supports the development of positive self-esteem for both the child and the parent."

"Theraplay is useful for a wide variety of children, including those who are withdrawn, depressed, over active, aggressive, have phobias or fine difficulty in socialising. Children with learning disabilities and developmental delays also benefit hugely from theraplay."

– Louise Shuttleworth, Psychotherapist, Clinical Partners UK

The mass behavioural problems with children are now no secret; social anxiety is almost the "new normal". Many teachers in schools are finding it hard to cope with all the non-academic issues they have to deal with. So knowing all that, why on earth would you completely shut off children from all their social activities? Schools closed, kids' clubs closed, whole families self-isolating in fear. Kids are being told to go completely against their natural instincts which are to physically play and chase and grab each other. I was working near a school when I saw about four young children in the school grounds playing in the bushes; they were about seven years old and having fun like kids do. I thought to myself, after such a long time since seeing this, *At, last kids playing normally*. Within about four minutes I heard a woman teacher's voice come over to them and shout, **"Keep away from each other and get out of there."**

It has been said that kids are more likely to die from lightning than "COVID". What on earth are we doing to our children's present and future mental health? A child with no issues will certainly struggle with this but imagine a child who has many difficulties in life; maybe school is the place where he/she can actually be free from stress for a while. What are the long-term consequences of people throwing their irrational fears onto children going to be?

The same reasoning can be given to adults with issues that were previously being dealt with through social meetings or therapies. Let's be clear, the consequences for mental health are going to be devastating and it is total nonsense to suggest that the people behind the lockdown would not know this. It will be interesting to see what the suicide rate for adults with mental health issues who are being locked down and socially isolated will be. This is mass torture and sadly, while the majority of the public are still being controlled through fear this time bomb is ticking and unless the Coronavirus Act is abandoned now and people are allowed to go out and socialise, it's only going to get worse. Kids going back to school now are actually being told not to hug their grandparents. And based on what? Well, as we have seen, it's not based on science.

Imagine being created to come into a world like that. Would you want to enter? Having no choice but to enter, would you want to pop out and enter the world with joy and excitement? Or do you think you may have already decided that this world is not for you and maybe your behaviours will reflect that in a way that we would call autistic?

Imagine for a minute the world children are being born and raised in now. What is their family environment like? What is the "new normal" at school like? What is their perception of the world? Is it a friendly place for adventure or a deadly place we need to survive?

This is complete madness.

THE WAR ON INFORMATION AND TRUTH

> "Every record has been destroyed or falsified, every book rewritten, every picture has been repainted, every statue and street building has been renamed, every date has been altered. And the process is continuing day by day and minute by minute. History has stopped. Nothing exists except an endless present in which the Party is always right."
>
> – George Orwell, *1984*

People who believe the myths spread by anti-vaccine campaigners **"are absolutely wrong"**, England's top doctor has said. Prof Dame Sally Davies said the MMR vaccine was safe and had been given to millions of children worldwide but uptake was currently **"not good enough"**. In England, 87% of children receive two doses but the target is 95%. The chief medical officer urged parents to get their children vaccinated and ignore **"social media fake news"**.

> "A number of people, stars, believe these myths – they are wrong," she said. "Over these 30 years, we have vaccinated millions of children. It is a safe vaccination – we know that – and we've saved millions of lives across the world. People who spread these myths, when children die they will not be there to pick up the pieces or the blame."

An interesting comment here would be that the UK has never achieved full measles herd immunity; 95% for at least the first two vaccines, but we haven't had the mass deaths they say would come back. They still push the fear but don't seem to be able to stop and question their own science.

Headlines like:

"Facebook fake news "war room" should target anti-vaxxers..."
– The Telegraph

"Half of new parents shown anti-vaccine misinformation on social media..."
– The Guardian

"MPs to investigate resurgence of anti-vaccine movement..."
– ITV news online

"Posting anti-vaccine propaganda on social media could become a criminal offence, Law Commissioner says..."
– The Telegraph

We have social media fact checkers warning us about posts and Facebook's own checkers blocking posts and YouTube removing people's channels for challenging vaccination and the current narrative on the corona pandemic. Add to this the 77th brigade with its thousands of people working behind the scenes and as the graphs have shown, it is clear the medical professionals themselves are being misinformed, then we really are in the middle of a war, a war of truth.

A good example is the Wales measles outbreak of 2013:

> "For the entire period 1 January to March 31, 2013 there were just 26 laboratory confirmed cases out of 446 notifications: 10 in January, 8 in February."
>
> "And in March just eight cases out of 302 notifications. That is a percentage rate of over-diagnosis and over-notification of 3774 %. Or put it another way 0.027 of notified cases were actually measles – and it is medical professionals who do the diagnosing and notifying. Kind of knocks your faith in the ability of doctors to diagnose a basic childhood illness. And we must not forget the poor man who died – but no one knows what he died of and three doctors did not diagnose it as measles."[33]

---

[33] https://www.informedparent.co.uk/uks-fake-welsh-measles-epidemic-only-8-cases-confirmed-for-march/

But if you were around at the time of the "outbreak" you will remember the media pushing out the fear propaganda, especially after the one death; though again, similar to today, it was a death "with" and not "of" and all that with an unreliable test. The media as usual push out the initial fear but when things calm down and the real figures come out they never go back and set things straight so the public are left with the great measles outbreak of Wales 2013 in their minds, the fear goes on and the control gets tighter.

Many whistle blowers, doctors, scientists and researchers who are putting their opinions out there for the public are now being censored or even banned from platforms like YouTube and Facebook and you will never see them on the BBC. But truth has to come out, and it will, as hard as they try; the more they censor, the more people question why. I'm not saying who is right or wrong. I have my opinion, yes, but what we need is a full, open debate for all the public to see. After any coup, control of information is the first thing that is done. Have we witnessed the "corona coup"?

THE SYSTEM

Human Sovereignty

The foundation of life for every human being is our individual God-given right over our own lives. This free will cannot be given or taken away by another man and is only yours to give up. Yes, there can be consequences of expressing your freedom sometimes but it is only your choice to be afraid that relinquishes your freedom. The only rule is to respect everyone else's sovereignty and "do no harm".

The Freeman Movement

Some people have decided to regain freedom and sovereignty by leaving man-made society. This is perfectly fine but they have to realise they cannot have any benefits of society anymore. They cannot even put litter in a public bin without paying for this service and if they get run over by a bus cannot even expect an ambulance unless willing to pay for the service. Even calling the police out to report a crime is not possible as all these things are not God-given but from man-made society. Freedom does, after all, have a price. It is still possible to live and work as normal, but as no membership of society equals no contributions, then no benefits can be expected either. It would also be possible to live as some have done in the wilderness as a hermit but in the book *Into the Wild* by Jon Krakauer, the young adventurer Christopher Johnson McCandless wrote in his diary shortly before his death in the Alaskan wilderness after years living on the road: **"Happiness only real when shared."**

Society

A "freeman" may enter society and create a membership with the creation of a "person" or identity. There are many ideas of what this "person" actually means and the late John Harris in his talk "It's an Illusion" found on YouTube is a good start. For me, it is just a membership of a society and an identity you can use to contract. So on entering a society – OK, so for the moment we have no choice – we are expected to contribute and receive benefits and adhere to the rules and regulations. Always remember, society is a man-made idea and its existence starts in our minds and then manifests into life; it is a manifestation of an idea, and as no man has authority over another it must be by consent.

It's clear that the creation of the birth certificate is your membership into society; this is how the **"person"** is created and the human being dies. By continuing to see ourselves as **"persons"** we are giving up our natural sovereignty and agreeing to live under the rules of the club. In theory common law should be our protection from a police state but in practice the government nowadays just make up laws as they go along and the police happily get on with enforcing them. The truth is, there is no option as to whether you should have a birth certificate, the decision has already been made and you WILL be part of society and live by its rules.

> Guardian Online, 23rd June, 2019:
>
> **"Man who refused to register son's birth loses high court case."**
>
> Judge: **"Hayden said the couple's deliberate decision not to register the birth stemmed from the boy's father's unusual and somewhat eccentric beliefs about the concept of personal sovereignty."**
>
> **"Mr Justice Hayden ruled the council had the right to step in as the child's "institutional parent" to register the birth."**
>
> **"The judge added the essence of the father's objection was "his belief that registration will cause his son to become controlled by a state which he perceives to be authoritarian and capricious."**
>
> **"He ruled: "It is manifestly in T's best interest for his birth to be registered, in order that he may be recognised as a citizen and entitled to the benefits of such citizenship."**

I wonder how many people now with what is going on and the coming crash of the world economy and all the COVID rules we have to follow, feel the benefit of being part of society, not to mention paying back the now over £2 trillion debt.

Public servants or leaders?

Let's be clear, those who work running society are public servants and not leaders, simple.

Have you noticed, though, over the last few years you don't really hear the words "public servants" anymore? It is all about our leaders. First, we are all our own leaders and this has to be understood. And next, what we should be worried about is, where are these leaders leading us to?

We need to start leading ourselves and start calling our public servants what they really are, **our servants.**

Compromise Yes, Conform No

For many different people to live freely and in peace in society there must sometimes be compromises. Not really any different from a marriage in that different people sometimes get into a situation where full agreement cannot be made, here reasonable compromises are needed so that things can move on and both parties feel at ease with the decision. What we should never do, though, is conform or allow ourselves to be forced into conforming to something that goes against all we believe to be true and right and against who we individually are.

Compromising can create peace and unity.

Conforming can create anger and division.

Just say NO

Learning to say **NO** is a powerful lesson on the road to self-empowerment. We need to learn to live and make decisions without being controlled by fear. Pick your battles at first, fight when you know you can win, leave hard battles for another day, know which battles are too important to leave and draw a line in the sand, stand firm and just say **NO.** Do not become a martyr for other people as self-empowerment is about changing yourself and nobody else. "Do not bite off more than you can chew," as they say.

A great philosophy on this is from Cesar Milan, famous as the "dog whisperer". He uses and teaches "calm, assertive energy" in all situations.

We need to take control of our own energy field to keep our minds clear and concentrated on the job; a deep breath when needed always helps. If we can all learn to say **NO** then bit by bit we can push forward to freedom and peace, just focus on yourself regardless of what others are doing as self-empowerment is only for you and with a bit of luck, if we all take this attitude and tend our own gardens then we can cultivate a paradise.

Society is just an expression of the collective thoughts and consciousness of the people in it; let's just sort out our own minds and lives and leave others to sort out theirs as they see fit. Give advice, yes, but in the end the only life you have a right to change is your own. Change society by changing yourself. **"Be the change you want to see in the world."**

Beware of anyone, especially in public service, who has a "vision" and wants to "change"; these people have an agenda which is about creating a world in their image. We are all different, and are also always changing, so any free society cannot be fixed or have a fixed destination.

> **"Speak your truth and don't invest in the outcome."**
> – Max Igan

Police State

Psychologist Jordan Peterson, a huge critic of Fascism and Marxism, has asked the question many times. Would you have taken part in taking people into the concentration camps and the gulags?

Almost all people say no. Yes, history tells us that almost all people do. Events are taking place now and policies are being passed as law that make it seem clear that history is about to repeat itself, only the concentration camps and gulags will be replaced by "quarantine centres".

Will you as a neighbour stand by and watch your family and friends taken away for "testing and surveillance"? Will you as police be the ones knocking down the doors and taking families away with children crying simple because a Public Health Officer suspects someone to be infected?

You cannot have a police state without the police working for the government. The police for now are confused about their role; they are here to protect the people and to keep the peace. They have now become enforcers of government policy and enemies of the truth, of the people and of freedom. If we can get the police on our side all this can be over very quickly and very peacefully. If not, I fear for the future. History does seem to be repeating itself.

It is said that we make all our decisions based on choosing the option that is closest to pleasure and the furthest away from pain. It seems then, that for many people true freedom is a very painful option and far away from pleasure, then slavery, whether conscious of it or not, is the furthest away from pain and closest to pleasure. It doesn't have to be pleasurable but it is better than the pain of true freedom and taking total responsibility for one's own life and true independence.

We need to stop voting for our own enslavement from my late friend, musical genius and long-time truther Ollie.

YouTube: **"Vote No More" directed and performed by Doc Mustard.**

FOLLOW THE MONEY

> "And Jesus went into the temple of God, and cast out all them that sold and bought in the temple, and overthrew the tables of the money changers, and the seats of them that sold doves, And said unto them, It is written, My house shall be called the house of prayer; but ye have made it a den of thieves."

Money is, or at least should be, a representation of our productive energies to be passed around to get around the problem of bartering. We may want something someone produces or a service they offer but we haven't got anything to exchange in return. So this little piece of paper (or now number on a computer) is exchanged, representing a certain agreed amount of my productive energies that can be redeemed at any time by anyone. Money being passed around is productive energies being passed around. The more you have of it, would fairly represent your productive output. The more money in circulation would indicate lots of productivity, and less money, less productive activity.

Just to be clear, everything we need in order to thrive has been given to us free by the creator. The sun doesn't charge us to come up every morning. Money is not a necessity to create wealth but just a tool to facilitate the fair passing of production. A fully conscious, compassionate, mankind could get on fine without it but that doesn't mean there is anything wrong with a monetary system providing it is being used fairly. So how is it being used?

In the UK at present over 97% of "money" comes into existence as credit/loans (new deposits). Most people think that when they deposit money in a bank, the bank then uses this same money to loan out to other people. Well, this couldn't be further from the truth. With factional reserve banking the bank only needs about 10% or even less in reserve, in deposits, to the amount it can loan. Meaning basically, when you get a loan from a bank the "money" they loan you is actually created out of thin air on a computer. Imagine this for a moment: you borrow £100,000 to buy a house and years later depending on interest rates you may pay back double and yet the bank never really loaned you anything. Yes, it was just created in five minutes on a screen and you slave away for years to pay back the interest. Not a bad hourly rate, I think you will agree! It is the document you sign which in fact creates this new money. You promise to pay with your future production, your working life.

This actually isn't the problem, creating money out of thin air. When you start to pay back your loan, you then take that money out of circulation as it was only put out there to represent your future earnings. The problem is the interest, because the bank only created the new money based on the amount of the loan, but they didn't create the interest. And when you see that interest charges now can range from 3% to over 1,000% on credit cards or payday loans, it becomes obvious that there is never enough money in circulation to pay back all the running loans. In fact, the only way the system can continue is with the constant introduction of "new deposits" in the form of more loans/debt. Watch on YouTube the documentary "Money as Debt".

Add to this that they can also sell this promise to play on the financial markets. We now have our credit being gambled on open markets and we all know what happened in 2008. Remember this when our highly paid alleged public servants tell us austerity is necessary because money doesn't grow on trees and they can't just create it out of thin air! Where do they actually think it comes from? If it isn't found in nature it has to have been created by men. This is a question you will never find being addressed by the corporate-controlled mainstream media or by our esteemed experts in parliament. This fact should now be more obvious with the massive furlough scheme, billions of pounds coming from nowhere when for years people have been homeless on the streets. This money, though, will be claimed back, and the holiday won't last forever.

One of the consequences of this is consumerism; the production of products, needed or not, to be made and passed through the conveyor belt for sale and to landfills as quickly as possible. So the insanity can continue to keep the debt-based system going. Try telling this to an environmental activist! This is what is causing environmental genocide. It would be wiser to campaign on the root of the problem than on the big corporations taking advantage of it.

This is why when the "experts" – nice suits from the City of London, an independent sovereign state within the UK like the Vatican within Italy – are interviewed on radio or television about the economy; they only talk about public consumer spending. Indeed, let us shop, shop, shop our way out of our financial problems. Highly paid, well educated, morons in braces, although I suspect some of them really know what they are doing! Even our own financial economic genius George Osbourne just talks about economic output and economic growth.

So tell me then, Mr Rishi Sunak, why exactly does the economy need to grow constantly? Why do you say immigration is great because of the amount they put into the economy? Yes, more consumers, another supporter of the economic plan to shop our way out of financial disaster.

The truth is it needs to grow to stop the whole system of debt collapsing, as we have already shown that there is never enough money in circulation to pay back all of the debt. And what happens when you can't pay your mortgage? We all know they come in and take the real wealth, which is the house. And when the banking system controls over 97% of money in circulation they can easily create booms and bust by just increasing or reducing the loans, which makes boom and bust organised theft. The present monetary system is an energetic drain on humanity. You get back a lot less in relation to what you put in and the men who control the system receive far more than they contribute. Come to think of it, they actually don't contribute anything. This is what this whole global corporate banking system is about, taking ownership (another man-made concept) of all the real wealth, like the World Bank and IMF are doing throughout the world and especially Africa and Latin America. I encourage you to read *The Open Veins of Latin America* by Eduardo Galeano. He talked about how the Spanish royalty may have taken over Latin America (the cow) but it was the bankers who took the riches (the milk). This present monetary system, and the people behind it, is responsible for not only our economic problems, but the wars, poverty, and environmental disasters on the planet.

Central Banks

The model for central banking is the Bank of England, again to be found in the sovereign state of the City of London. It was formed by subscribers to fund the rebuilding of the British Navy after the war. Subscribers were lending money to the British Government providing the nation's finances were handed over to them to handle. So it started out as a private bank in the old way of the Court Jews, facilitating loans on behalf of the government. They now control interest rates and are told to keep inflation below about 2% though there doesn't seem to be any consequence if they don't. They hold the reserves of the high street banks. Basically a private bank paid to borrow money from other private banks and corporations to enslave the host nation into an unpayable debt. Yes, the present Bank of England has been nationalised, but that just means basically that the government bought up all the shares.

In the case of the Federal Reserve in the USA it is totally owned by private banks and yes, you guessed it, founded in the sovereign state of the District of Colombia, together with its close friends the IMF and the World Bank. What is important is the function of the bank and not who owns it. And its function is to facilitate debt and control (manipulate) interest rates. This surely constitutes a conflict of interest. **"No man can serve two masters for he will either hate the one and love the other, or else he will hold to the one."** – Mathew 6:24.

Look at the world's economic problems and where the wealth is going and decide who the master of these central bankers is. Also, have a look on the websites of central banks and the IMF, World Bank and the Bank of International settlements, founded in "neutral" Switzerland, and all you see is corporate talk, including one thing they all have in common which is privatisation. Their loans have stipulations like having to privatise your water supply and as these loans cannot be paid back, the debt is bigger than the loan, they will then go into debt slavery and forced privatisation to just pay off the loans. All a big scam!

Enough of the problem, though, now to solutions.

Glass Steagall

In the US, the Banking Act of 1933, commonly known as the Glass Steagall Act, stated "the separation of commercial and investment banking", which prevented security firms and investments banks from taking deposits and commercial Federal Reserve member banks from dealing in non-governmental securities for customers, which otherwise could lead them to invest in non-investment-grade securities for themselves, underwriting or distributing non-governmental securities affiliating (or sharing employees) with companies involved in such activities.

Easily put, separate the criminal gambling from our day-to-day banking so those of us who choose not to gamble with our hard-earned money will not be affected by those who do. This will remove enormous power from the criminal bankers and gamblers, making money from money and making money from debt in what is in fact a big worldwide casino. This is an absolutely necessary first step towards a just monetary system and only complete separation, not George Osbourne's "ring fence", will do the trick. Criminals always find ways of getting round or under fences.

The myth of a gold-backed currency

Many now are putting forward a gold-backed currency to stabilise the financial system. Again, I will be brief and recommend Bill Still again and his documentary on YouTube, "The Secret of OZ", for a full understanding of why gold is not a good idea.

Firstly, who owns all the gold?

We know Gordon Brown sold off half the UK gold reserves at a rock-bottom price, without asking us. It is now mainly in the hands of private banks and investors and not in Fort Knox, as Bill Still points out. So again, we gave the criminal bankers the control.

Next, does this mean that when a country has no gold it will remain poor forever, subjected to the will of the "gold merchants"? Will we then see wars over gold reserves and more poor African and Latin American nations being commercially invaded by corporate military, if need be, to control gold mining?

Next, economists say we need a gold-backed currency as it controls the amount of money in circulation which prevents inflation. These "experts" simply do not understand that the amount of money in circulation isn't what causes inflation; it is the amount of money in relation to productivity that causes inflation. Little productivity and lots of money equals inflation, hence why Quantitative Easing does not work as it has no backing, it is just printing money in hopes of stimulating the economy. As long as money is backed by and represents productivity there will be no inflation. Controlling the money supply only controls growth. And surely we don't want to control growth! Bringing money into circulation based on productivity and taken out when productivity is low creates stability.

Last, people who put forward a gold-backed currency have lost sight of what true wealth is. It cannot be found in so-called precious metals that cannot be used to feed us or clothe us or keep us warm. We are the wealth, our ideas and productivity using the resources available to us. The resource in itself is not the wealth as without our imagination and human work it doesn't do anything, provides us with nothing. Give a starving man a choice of a table full of gold and a table full of food and he knows only the food will sustain him.

A just monetary system for all

So if we go back to money just being a representation of productivity founded on creative ideas and natural resources, then here is my model for a fair and just system.

Stop government borrowing NOW.

Bring in complete Glass Steagall separation of investment and commercial banking. This will also allow us to stop bailing out banks. No more bailouts. Let them fail. Direct from the treasury produce our own credit, based on what we need to produce as a nation: fiscal expenses, to go on roads, infrastructure, schools, healthcare, transport and energy.

Nationalise the basic things of life to maintain society, such as utilities, water and energy, roads, and main transport routes. In my opinion schools and healthcare are not such a simple area to nationalise as enormous changes need to be made first. Currently they are not being run for the benefit of the people and people should always have a choice of healthcare and education. I would suggest, though, having a national accident and emergency department.

Ban all interest on loans. Introduce an upfront regulated service charge as a fee for extending credit. Then only the amount credited is to be paid back. This means the service charge will come out of the present existing money supply, so when the new money/credit is being created there will always be enough money in circulation to pay back the loan. The money that is created by the treasury is interest-free and the only debt attached to its use would be in the building of roads, the supplying of energy and other things the money was produced for in the first place. The debt will be in making excellent use of the credit given, so it's a debt of creating more, like more jobs and more wealth. Basically, anything we can imagine, we can produce the money needed to manifest it. Hence, this would be a great time to invest in real science and engineering and a great time to pursue free energy.

I don't advocate a total ban on fractional reserve banking, as some suggest. Just as it is not good when the banking system has almost total control of the money supply; it would equally not be a good idea to let the government have all the control. Always spread the power out.

A well-regulated system where the banks can create credit for private businesses and people, where the borrower and lender are held responsible for the new money being productive, can work well. We don't want to go into a Communist-style money system with total government control. This is the failing of the Cuban Revolution. Yes, they kicked out the banks and international corporations but they also took over everything and took away the people's right to lead their own lives and run their own businesses. Extreme socialism is an ideal that can never work as individuals have different dreams and they aspire to different things. With the recent economic changes in Cuba it seems they are waking up to this reality.

Going from George Orwell, "All men are born lazy but some are lazier than others," why should one man work hard whilst the other is not and still receive the same in rewards? We need motivation, inspiration and incentive to work hard and create and manifest our ideas and the pursuit of material gain is not wrong in itself.

Keeping available credit away from government allows us to imagine and manifest our ideas and pursue personal economic freedom, not depending on big government to provide all our needs. That, in the end, is disempowering. We are searching for self-empowerment and self-reliance, with only the backup of the state when needed. These steps will put an end to the insane destruction of the environment and real sustainability and working in harmony with nature can be realised when people locally are allowed to deal with the issues surrounding their land.

No debt will also mean less time spent working to pay off debt and more time spent enjoying family life, dreaming and pondering the wonders of the universe.

Does this mean an end to taxation? No; taxation will be used to control the amount of money in circulation, so that it is in relation to production. Taking money out of circulation when productivity is low helps prevent inflation and enables a steady, balanced economy. Taxation gain can then be re-invested into new production and any shortfall for big projects can just be created again, instead of borrowing again. The amount of money in circulation should always represent the amount of productive activity.

At the moment there is plenty of work to be done but, in the present system, they say, not enough money to fund it. Well, for God's sake, create it! Interest-free credit, backed by the ideas we want to manifest, means any idea or productivity can be made to manifest simply by producing the money to facilitate it. The needed work dictates the money supply and not the other way round.

With the UK Government debt now passing £2 trillion and interest payments alone over £1 billion per week and add to that the mortgage debt, credit cards, private loans and the pension pot black hole, it must be very clear that as a nation we are bankrupt; in fact the whole of the western world is and we may as well include the rest of the planet too. This debt has not come about by accident and the fact we are all bankrupt is because of policies or stupid economists working for government. It is deliberate policy designed to crash a system so they can bring in a one-world solution. This is why I support the UK Column[34] and their campaign for national credit in the form of the treasury-produced Bradbury pound.

Beware the Gobal Reset – World Economic Forum

The well-documented problem-reaction-solution has its fingerprints all over this pandemic. (World Economic Forum – event 201) Since the 2008 financial crash when the governments bailed out banks instead of people it has been well known the system itself was not fixed and that even before the pandemic we were already on the verge of the biggest financial crash in history.

Do you think the people would allow the same thing to happen again? I don't think so. This pandemic, the lockdown and the organised destruction of the world economy cannot be by accident, these people are not that stupid. On the surface maybe but this is very organised and controlled. People are not already expecting a massive financial crash and will probably be happy enough to blame it on the "virus" even when they are losing their jobs, home, freedom and future.

The reconstruction of how we do business and how we exchange money has already been planned with a heavy slant on "the green economy". Basically there will be a certain way to do business and if you don't follow the regulations then you will fail, and this is coming from the central

---

[34] www.ukcolumn.org

bankers who control the world and not from the people themselves. The reset is just about total control and we need to be careful not to fall into the trap no matter how well it is sold to us.

Control means they have to get rid of cash so when they announced the "virus" spreading on cash that at least did give me a laugh that day, even with all the madness going on around.

I'm pretty sure Bill gates and his 060606 patent and ID 2020 will be involved somehow.

Still not convinced of the control the international banks have over our country? Here is a letter from the Rothschild bank to **"The Rt Hon George Osborne MP, Chancellor of the Exchequer"** dated **10th June 2015, regarding "The government's shareholding in the Royal Bank of Scotland".**[35]

> **"You asked us to provide you with an assessment of whether or not it is appropriate and in the interests of taxpayers for the government to start to sell its stake in the Royal Bank of Scotland Group plc (RBS). This document summarises the analysis we have undertaken and sets out our resulting conclusions."**
>
> **"… we believe that it is now in the interest of taxpayers for the government to set in train an initial small disposal of RBS shares for a number of reasons."**

So George Osbourne, whose position in the Treasury you would expect means he would be an expert in economics, had written to the Rothschild bank, a private bank, for advice for the selling of shares in a bank that was bailed out by the British Government, without permission of the people and taxpayers they claim to serve, to solve a problem created by international bankers in the first place. Their advice was to start to sell and what did he do?

On the 4th August 2015, the government began the sale of its shares in the Royal Bank of Scotland, selling at a loss, 5.4% @330p a share, raising £2.1 billion.

---

[35]
https://assets.publishing.service.gov.uk/government/uploads/system/uploads/attachment_data/file/434155/
Rothschild_letter_to_the_Chancellor.pdf

And where did that £2.1 billion go?

To pay off the fraudulent government debt.

In other words, straight back into the hands of the big banks and corporations who created the mess in the first place.

On the government website they claim that they paid off the "national debt" with the income from the sale but I'm not so sure as that would include private debt and I don't remember receiving any income from the government to pay off any of my private debt. This does, though, go to show that the Treasury themselves, or the humans that work there, don't even know the difference between National and Government debt; they really are clueless, at least on the surface.

This is just a rundown of the criminal debt-based money system, and doesn't even go into the multi billions that the drug and vaccine industry make every year. The mind boggles at how much a COVID-19 vaccine will make. Think of around seven billion people having probably at least two shots and maybe every year, we are talking trillions. Maybe Bill Gates has a good investment after all.

We do, though, have a historic precedent in dealing with these people and the example of Jesus showed us what is needed. Time to turn over the tables of the money changers!

WHAT NEXT?

"It is no measure of health to be well adjusted to a profoundly sick society."

– J Krishnamurti

Humanity is now at a crossroads and this sure does seem the time for the final battle of Good vs Evil. The true battle is a battle for our minds, our beliefs, for it is those beliefs that will control our behaviour. The real battle then is for consciousness or awareness, for if we are being controlled by beliefs we have no conscious knowledge of, then how can we free ourselves? Becoming conscious is the first step.

Yes, we lived in a profoundly sick society, all of us; a sickness that has infected all nations, all cultures and all people. We, humanity, are out of balance. To restore balance individually and collectively we need to become conscious, conscious of who we are, of our actions and how they affect others. Most of the world are living semi-conscious or unconscious lives, indoctrinated to act or think a certain way by a system that isn't even real, by organised religion and belief systems that serve to imprison the spirit of man. We identify with our nationality, but even that is a man-made idea (try saying that to the cultural Marxists trying to put countless identities on all of us in the name of freedom).

What we are, all are, are sovereign human beings, we have just forgotten, helped by our controllers who want us to forget. True balance is expressing the fullness of who you are, your true self, in harmony with your surroundings and respecting every other expression of self under the universal law of "do no harm". When you cannot be yourself, whether it is because of indoctrinated belief systems, oppressive regulations of society, or fear of being different then you cannot truly be in balance.

Fearful, indoctrinated minds create a "survival of the fittest" mentality leading to wars and violent behaviour, and just in case people start to "wake up" we have the endless distractions to divert our attention. The search for the true self means throwing away all that is false; like looking for a needle in a haystack, throw out what is not the needle and eventually what is left must be the needle.

Belief systems must go as they create limitations. A realisation that no man has authority over another is a must. Understand that we are all different expressions of self; there is no one-size-fits-all, and look to nature to guide you too, as nature always looks to be in balance. And also accepting that our life is our own we cannot expect or insist that everyone else has to "wake up"; the only person that needs to change is you as you have authority over yourself and no-one else.

We are spiritual beings having a human experience, **that is it**, nothing else to learn, just to unlearn and then express your true self. As far as we know we have one shot at life and we are just throwing it away obeying orders from psychopaths in a shirt and tie.

By taking control of our thoughts and beliefs, understanding our own God-given sovereignty, accepting responsibility for our own lives, being our own leaders, being reasonable, making compromises, not conforming, using common sense, learning to say NO and accepting that your idea of what is right for you may not be right for others, if this leads to self-empowerment then yes, we can have Freedom, or something like that.

Lose the fear of authority. **"And fear not them which kill the body, but are not able to kill the soul: but rather fear him which is able to destroy both soul and body in hell."** – Matthew 10:28.

We are all energy. Energy cannot be destroyed; the body is our vehicle for this experience and it has a life span, it's going back to dust anyway. We have a choice. We can live a long life in fear and with our heads bowed down and then die having not really lived, or we can stand up straight and look them all in the eye and live life as we see fit, and if they put us against a wall and point the rifles then just look them in the eyes and laugh. Our body was going to die anyway and now it's just the end of the game. We go back to your source, and there is no council tax there. As Bill Hicks says, **"it's just a ride"**.

> **"The meaning of life is just to be alive. It is so plain and so obvious and so simple. And yet, everyone rushes round in a great panic as it were necessary to achieve something beyond themselves."**
>
> – Alan Watts

Patrick Quanten, in his search of true health and understanding of disease eventually brought everything down to one simple thing, **self-empowerment.** At his website you can learn through his videos and his paper "The Missing Science in Medicine" and more articles on how to take over the decision making in your own life. That really is the foundation for freedom and health, and if we are all free to make our own decisions then individually all decisions are valid and everyone can just get on, living a life they choose to live but also taking responsibility for those choices also.[36]

Action

The pen is mightier than the sword

Of course creating awareness is the major thing that needs to be done, for without understanding the nature of the problems we are facing we will never find any real solutions and will be led down a pathway that will enslave us into the "prison without walls" so expertly described in Huxley's *Brave New World* with the "Orwellian" jackboot for those of us who do not wish to comply. We can all research this stuff and talk to our families and neighbours, even talking in the now communist-style queues whenever we go shopping.

But one of the main reasons to write this booklet was to give the ordinary man or woman the information to start to challenge those who claim authority over our decision making. The graphs are simple to understand and can be copied and sent to MPs, doctors, nurses, teachers, councillors and the like. The simple lie about the nature of fluoride can easily be challenged. The information on smallpox can be used to challenge the basis for all vaccination programmes. Letters can even be signed "a concerned parent" or "a worried citizen" so you don't feel threatened.

One thing is for sure, doing nothing is not an option. I asked Mike Robinson of the UK Column many years ago after time spent under the radar, "What are the consequences of doing what I need to do?"

He just told me, "What are the consequences of doing nothing?"

The answer is simple and there is no choice; doing nothing is not an

---

[36] https://www.pqliar.net/

option. What you do as an individual in your own personal circumstances is up to you; with the information here anyone is able to write an anonymous letter.

CHALLENGE – START SAYING NO – WITHDRAW CONSENT

Support and watch the UK Column.

Two women that have inspired me to keep speaking my truth:

Allona Lahn, part of the "Informed medical Objections Party" in Australia:

> "I talk LOUD because I love my family, I talk because I want a better future for everyone, I talk because MASS DRUGGING is now the norm and we have a very sick society and I can see in the future the mass health issues we are creating. Everyone should be concerned about the future and just how many drugs you and your family will be coerced into having. I suggest EVERYONE support me and those that question the billion $$ pharmaceutical industry, you see it will be us that creates a better society, better health care system, sustainable communities and a Healthier World… because we are demanding truth, transparency and a healthier, natural, safer healthcare system and drugs!
>
> LET'S HAVE THE DISCUSSION I'm keen…"

And Magdaline Taylor of The Informed Parent.[37]

> An Educated Decision
>
> "More and more parents are questioning the safety and effectiveness of vaccinations. Greater knowledge enables parents to have the confidence to exercise their right to an informed choice. At The Informed Parent we think you are entitled to a wide spectrum of information that will help you make up your own mind."

Whether you believe viruses are the cause of disease or the result of disease is up to you. All I am asking for is an open public scientific debate

---

[37] https://www.informedparent.co.uk/

from both sides.

We still have one question to answer. **Do you want to be free?**

If we are all free to choose, whether we choose to be afraid and isolate or to just get on with life, to accept a vaccine or not, to choose to wear a mask or not, it has to come from us. The system does not provide a choice. We have to start to learn to live outside of the system if we cannot change it.

In the UK and the Commonwealth we have a system of common law based on human sovereignty that could be used to bring back freedom to the people and fix a broken system. If that fails, though, we need to start to think for ourselves and try to find a life in our own "bubble" existence within a society we cannot totally leave. As no one knows the future then it certainly is a great time to really live in the now because the now is all that we can guarantee. The world has officially gone mad and I want to get off, but I can't, I'll have to stick it out like the rest.

Positive thinking may open doors of opportunity but only positive action walks through them. With our backs now against the wall and nowhere to go, it's time to stand up and face what is in front of us. Brian Gerrish of the UK Column did that many years ago and has been a major force trying to expose child abuse at the highest level and the dark agenda it connects to.

It's now a spiritual battle

When the first lockdown was announced last year I was at karate club with the kids and talking to a friend who is "awake". She asked me, "Is it time to panic?"

My reply was, "No, it's time to go home and have a cup of tea."

The years of trying to warn people, the highs and lows, anger, frustration, disappeared at once; the battle had now begun. Like a boxer who has gone through all of the emotions during training, when he enters the ring it all goes away and he is just in the moment.

I have been really laid back now this last year and as things got worse, fascism wise, over the new year, I went to bed for a couple of days and realised that I no longer have any power at all, not even to protect my home and my family. As my friend and fellow Mancunian and

Wythenshawe lad James O'Neil and author of *Meg's Absolutely Wonderful Tremendous Fantastic Day/The Deafening Silence* always tells me, "God has all the power." Yes, he was right. From being laid back the last year it was time to let any illusion of control over my life to rest. It was now all in the hands of "God", "the Universe", "the Creator", or whatever. It was also a big relief as there was simply no, point in worrying about things totally out of my control.

Whatever the nature of the battle going on at this moment on Planet Earth, it's way beyond me as an individual. I still have a part to play but my part is a lot clearer than before. In the story of Jesus in The Bible what did he do that struck such fear into people that they had him killed?

Speak the truth.

Expose the lie.

Show compassion and empathy.

Kick out the money lenders.

Whatever your personal understanding is of life and creation, the battle of Good vs Evil, Light vs Darkness, Truth vs Lie, we have to move forward with connection to the energy that created us. Political rallies have proven, again, to solve nothing, especially if they are just childish tantrums from people who are just shouting for better terms of their enslavement. Sadly these well-meaning people can't see the true scale of the problem we are facing. Any actions now have to have a foundation of spiritual connection and we have to allow ourselves to be guided.

Most people are waiting for some kind of normality so they can get on with their lives. In reality, this would let the people behind this evil off the hook again as the population will be so glad of normality they will not even begin to challenge and hold to account their glorious leaders. Let this be the final battle and the end of the war on humanity; the more they push, the more they will force us into a corner and the more people will resist. It is gonna be very difficult, especially for those not wanting to confront Truth and Evil and wanting to hold on to a system that has enslaved them. But there is nowhere to go, nowhere to run and nowhere to hide.

James also says "never underestimate evil", which is why many of the decent people on the planet cannot comprehend the things going on around them, they simply cannot even imagine the evil that is taking place therefore it's dismissed from their minds, even though they can see it happening in front of them, a kind of cognitive dissonance. The world has been filled with darkness for a very long time; there is no saviour outside of yourself. As the Hopi Indians have stated, "we are the ones we've been waiting for", or as my friend Patrick Quanten says, "the only light at the end of the tunnel or in it is the light you shine yourself".

Take a deep breath, connect to whatever creation is, be guided and remember, positive thinking has to be backed up by positive action.

Hold tight, start shining, it's gonna be a bumpy ride.

> **"We have no choice to be in the world. The only choice we have is how we respond to the fact that we live in the world."**
> – Yolande Norris-Clark

> **"When one can see no future, all one can do is the next right thing."**
> – Frozen 2

What a crazy world we live in – maybe David Icke is not mad after all.

THE BEST CHICKEN SOUP EVER!

End of summer 1998. Mission: fly to New York and somehow, some way, get to Rio for the millennium. Just a few hundred quid, a dream and knowing it was now or never. I was gonna eat the best food, drink the best beer and have all the adventures on the way, yes, and with just that few hundred quid. How was I gonna do it? I didn't know. Was I gonna survive? I didn't care. It just had to be done, man against the world.

New York, Miami, Texas and all in between; great times, great people but now to cross the border into strange lands and unknown possibilities. Crossing the border into Mexico at midnight, the only white man on the bus and I was stopped by the American police. *What is this little white English guy doing here?* they must have thought. After pulling me to one side and making sure I wasn't a mass murderer on the run they let me pass. Now I was here, over the border into new territory.

Two men approach and ask me if I need a hotel. One a taxi driver, one a policeman. I roll the dice and go with the policeman; at least he said he was gonna take me round the corner. The taxi driver, well, who knows where he would have taken me? I pulled out my main form of protection, a Manchester United souvenir, a scarf. We talked about David Beckham, made friends and ten minutes later I was in a hotel, door shut, locked and safe.

The next morning in the light I walked out into this strange new land and the real adventure started now. Six weeks later I left Mexico, after eating maybe the best street food on Earth, some nice cold beers with lime in them – come to think of it most things were served with limes.

Venezuela for the South American tour. After a few days in Caracas I met up with Andy, another lad from northern England who I had met in Miami. We had arranged to keep in touch and we met up in Caracas so he could join in the adventure. Just a few days later on a ship to a Caribbean island we met Dave from Australia, later to become Crocodili Dave, at the bar of course, and over a couple of beers he was sold. We had a new recruit; we were now the "Three Amigos".

We ate all the food and washed it down with all the beer. We walked and slept on the ground through savanna land with snakes and scorpions for company. We climbed mountains, swam in piranha-infested waters and met all the weird and wonderful people along the way. We got stuck in Manaus in the heart of the Amazon, part by choice and part because we couldn't get a boat to get us out, always "we sail tomorrow", so another night on the beer then, another day of eating "meat-like" burgers. You could get it all – crocodile burger, piranha soup, turtle soup, insect and grubs on a stick, but no bat soup so far.

Then eventually we sadly said goodbye to Manaus, in a village river boat for four nights down the Rio Madeira. The boat was crammed, animals and helpers below and the rest of us on deck. Sardines in a can when all the hammocks were out at night. Eating rice and beans twice a day after a breakfast of tea and bread, the cooking water coming straight out of the murky river below and showering in the same water – the same water the sewage just went into.

On the first day Andy got the fever, the Latin lady eye fever; one look and he was gone like Mowgli walking into the man village, and four more nights crammed up in a hammock under the romantic Amazon moon and we lost him.

We got off after four days and then after a 36-hour bus journey through the Brazilian Amazon we got off in a town somewhere. I am not sure where exactly but I am sure it was somewhere, it must have been somewhere because we were there. We stayed the night and after a meal and another few beers and a good night's sleep we left Andy with his eyes still hypnotised and fully infected.

So now there were two.

A few days later we made it to Rio, New Year's Eve morning. Copacabana was too expensive for us, millennium prices, so we took two buses four hours out of town to a beach camping ground then four hours back to the Copacabana. We made it, just two hours to go but somehow, some way, we were there and ten minutes later Andy arrived too. He said he would be there and he was good to his word. One last fling with boys to finish what we had started, together.

Champagne and many beers later and well into the next morning, we were all lost, split up and in different parts of Rio. I got back to the tent somehow about seven in the morning, David a couple of hours behind, Andy, well, he never made it back and that was the last we saw of him, he had Latin love on his mind. So it was me and Dave again.

Many places, adventures, rivers, mountains, deserts and even an illegal Bolivian prison tour later we were in La Paz, the cheapest place so far on our trip. We were planning more trips and more street food and much more beer for our next leg up to the north to cross the Atacama into Peru.

After all the plans were set, we were set to leave La Paz for the next leg. There we were outside a bus station, life everywhere, sitting on the floor, wild dogs looking for scraps – they probably peed where we were just sitting, diesel fumes everywhere from buses, taxis and wagons. The noise, the life, the culture, the dirt, and the middle-aged plump Bolivian lady in her traditional dress of layered skirts, cardigan and bowler hat, her hands as rough and as dirty as mine. On the floor was a big pot with steam coming out, her tin bowls and a big pot of murky soapy water to "clean" the dishes and some homemade "juice" in a plastic jug, no hand sanitiser in sight. We couldn't resist. We'd had a few beers the night before, well, that's how we made our plans, and had a long bus ride ahead. Two bowls of that hot chicken soup were ordered and a glass of that "juice". She served it while her baby boy was suckling on her breast, breast milk even pouring out of his nose as he couldn't get it down quick enough. We got stuck in; hot soup fresh made, where I don't know but I'm sure it was fresh where she made it. Incredible flavour and all natural, even had a hint of cream, or was it some breast milk that had slipped from the little boy's nose and into the bowl? Well, who cares? It tasted great and after a night on the beer was just what we needed to set us on our way for the next adventure.

We drank all the beer, the jungle juice too, all the street food, the good, the bad, and the ugly, and met some crazy people on the way. Some dodgy toilets, some without even toilet roll so we used our imagination, sometimes the odd bush, but we did it and we knew what it was like to be free, to experience the roller-coaster ride of life, but as we wanted.

And twenty years later we are all still here to tell the tale. Apart from a few times when we had to run to the toilet – well, even our bodies had their limits – we were alive, strong and well until I too got "infected" in Peru and left Dave to go on alone.

How on earth did we survive?

Danger everywhere, dodgy food and dodgy beer, in dodgy bars, sleeping in dodgy hotels. Not that South America is all like that but they are the places we chose to frequent. We wanted to see and experience the real life of the real people. To live surrounded by dirt and disease, dodgy toilets, "meat-like" burgers, real working people full of life and life's struggles. The hard life in South America means most people live for the day, whereas most westerners strive to be in "the now". To be free, to experience life, the now is all most of them have.

We survived all that and lived to tell the tale. Apart from the odd day rushing to the toilet, or the odd bush, we survived. We survived because we were three young men on an adventure, we were just passing through, we came into their world with all their dangers but we were just visiting. We didn't have to live the life there, the social, economic, cultural and political life that was making them poor. The polluted environment for them became an extra burden they couldn't take; we just seemed to shrug it off. We didn't succumb to their diseases, just the odd day running to the toilet. We ate the "meat-like" burger and we never set off a global pandemic. We didn't eat bat soup, not that we know of, but we survived and the world survived too.

As for Andy, well, his "infection" wore off, they sometimes do.

Dave, well, he got "bitten" somewhere in Asia.

As for me, well, twenty years and three kids later, let's face it, it's terminal.

There is more to life than the system, and there is more to disease than dirt. Life is a balance of all and more than everything an adventure to be lived. More should have our adventures and know real freedom, if only for a while, then maybe what is really making us sick in this world will become more obvious.

I thank Nature, or God, for all the adventures I had, for the people I met, and the lessons I learnt.

But most of all I thank God for that woman outside the Bolivian bus station (and her son) for just when we needed it most, serving up the best chicken soup, EVER.

Rob Ryder
May 2021

Printed in Great Britain
by Amazon